Overcoming Common Problems

Treating Arthritis
The drug-free way

Margaret Hills, SRN

Fourth edition revised by
Christine Horner, ECNP

sheldon **PRESS**

This book is dedicated to my family, without whom I might have given up the fight and succumbed, in self-pity, sentencing myself to a life of excruciating pain and immobility. So, to my husband, Ivan, and our children, Michael, Christine, Graham, Sally, Clive, Peter, William and Mary, thank you.

First published in Great Britain in 1985

Sheldon Press
36 Causton Street
London SW1P 4ST
www.sheldonpress.co.uk

Second edition published 1994
Third edition published 2004
Fourth edition published 2012

British Library Cataloguing-in-Publication Data
A catalogue record for this book is available from the British Library

ISBN 978–1–84709–237–3
eBook ISBN 978–1–84709–238–0

Typeset by Fakenham Prepress Solutions, Fakenham, Norfolk NR21 8NN
Printed in Great Britain by Ashford Colour Press
Subsequently digitally printed in Great Britain

eBook by Fakenham Prepress Solutions, Fakenham, Norfolk NR21 8NN

Produced on paper from sustainable forests

Contents

About the authors

The late Margaret Hills, SRN, trained at St Stephen's Hospital, London. She developed osteoarthritis and rheumatoid arthritis as a young woman, but went on to finish her nurse's training, marry, have eight children and pursue a long career as an industrial nurse. She developed her own method of natural treatment for arthritis and ran a clinic in Kenilworth. The clinic, now run by her daughter Christine Horner, attracts patients from far and wide and, following on from its success, Margaret wrote this book to impart her knowledge and help people with arthritis everywhere.

Christine Horner, ECNP, is a Nutritional Medicine practitioner and, having gained practical experience working alongside Margaret for many years, was able to continue the work of the Clinic on her mother's retirement. Safe, effective pain relief is invaluable in helping people with arthritis and modern technology plays an important role in this field: Scenar, InterX, low-level laser and the therapeutic blanket are all sophisticated therapies in which Christine has trained to support the dietary and nutritional supplements that are an essential part of the Clinic protocol for arthritis.

Preface

In September 1946, at the age of 21, I started training as a nurse at St Stephen's Hospital, Fulham Road, London. I was fun-loving and carefree; I loved to dance, cycle and swim, and my greatest ambition was to be a good nurse.

During the first year things went wonderfully well, and I began to love my chosen career. Discipline was very strict and the work was hard, but the rewards made it all worthwhile. Early in April 1947, I began to feel unwell. The doctor diagnosed acute rheumatoid arthritis and I was confined to the nurses' sick bay. Here it was discovered that I had a very enlarged heart and I was ordered complete rest, unable to wash or feed myself. A Harley Street heart specialist was consulted and he came every other day to examine my heart, while my progress was noted daily by the Medical Superintendent.

At this time, I was suffering extreme pain and discomfort. I was being nursed between blankets and because I could not bear the weight of the bedclothes, I had a cradle to protect my painful limbs. For four months I lay in bed, totally helpless; then gradually, I was allowed to sit out of bed, and to wash and feed myself. The only treatment I received, apart from complete rest, was aspirin. In those days, there were none of the drugs for arthritis that are available today.

After five months, I was allowed home to convalesce. Before leaving the hospital, the Medical Superintendent came to see me. 'Now my dear,' he said, 'you have been very ill, and your heart has been badly enlarged, so I must tell you that you must never dance or cycle again. You must not run uphill, or upstairs, and you must not come back to finish your nurse's training – the work is far too taxing. Also, if you ever marry, you must not have children. Last, but not least, be prepared for recurrences.'

As I walked out of the hospital gates, I thought, 'If I am to live my life like this, I may as well be dead.' I resolved there and then to do what I wanted, when I wanted, and not to tell my parents of the advice that I had been given. I had put on weight, owing to swelling of the tissues caused by my enlarged heart and also to inactivity from lying in bed for four months. I had gone from a trim nine stone six pounds to eleven stone three pounds, and I took a size seven shoe instead of size six. Nevertheless, I adopted a 'don't care' attitude, and I was determined to enjoy any time that I had left. So I danced, cycled and swam at every opportunity, soon losing the excess weight that I had gained. At the end of three months, I was quite surprised to find that I was still alive.

I still desperately wanted to become a nurse, so I wrote to the Matron at St Stephen's. I asked if I might resume my training as I was now feeling quite well. Imagine my delight when she agreed – so back I went.

By this time, I had developed osteoarthritis and from time to time suffered great pain. However, I managed to get through my training, and on passing my finals was placed in the operating theatre as Staff Nurse. This was the hardest job in the hospital, but I loved the work and was determined to live each day at a time. I felt that at least I had realized my first ambition – to be a fully trained nurse.

My second ambition, to get married, was to be realized the following year, when I met my husband. I left St Stephen's, moved to Coventry, where my husband worked, and obtained a job as an Industrial Nurse. However, it was not long before we started a family, and I left work.

Unfortunately, I was now suffering from chronic osteoarthritis, which often caused me great pain. I had always hoped that some day, somehow, it would go away, but it gradually got worse and worse. Sixteen years and six children later, I had another bout of rheumatoid arthritis, which left me totally crippled – locked in every joint.

By then, arthritic drugs had invaded the market. I went to see a well-known specialist in the treatment of arthritis, who duly prescribed a 'wonder drug'. However, when my panel doctor heard of this, he informed me that two recent deaths had been attributed to it and advised me to take it only when the pain was very bad. I was already taking 12 aspirins a day for the pain, so I tried to manage with these, since I considered them to be less dangerous, with fewer side-effects.

By now I was forced to wear a surgical collar, splints on my deformed fingers, a surgical corset and built-up arches for my shoes.

My consultant advised me to obtain a wheelchair. My experience in hospital had made me realize that the medical profession could do nothing for my arthritis. With six young children and a husband to look after, with very little money to pay for a home help, and with myself totally crippled and unable to move without excruciating pain, the future indeed looked bleak.

I have always believed in the saying, 'The Lord helps those who help themselves', so I prayed, then set out to research a cure for myself. I got hold of all the 'natural cure' books that I could lay my hands on, and eventually hit upon the treatment that was to rid me of all signs of arthritis in just 12 months and that has kept me totally pain-free since. Necessity really is the 'mother of invention', and the necessity was certainly there. My nurse's training, and the knowledge of the human body that I had acquired during that training, helped me to develop – from many combined ideas collected from the research that I had done – the treatment and diet with which I have had so much personal success over the years and with which there has been much wider success in my busy Clinic.

I hope that passing on my knowledge to readers of this book will help to relieve some of the pain of arthritis that is so prevalent among young and old alike, in practically every country in the world today. Since being published, this book has been translated into several languages and is on sale in several countries throughout the world. I never thought for a moment that it would bring so much relief to so many. Day after day, the letters arrive from people in various countries telling me how much they have benefited from following the treatment described within its pages and thanking me for writing it. I feel so humble and grateful when I learn that somebody, somewhere, whom I have never seen, feels better because of something I have done.

I opened the Margaret Hills Clinic in 1982 and it has gone from strength to strength. We now treat over 800 people at any given time. Consultations at the Clinic are held daily. Needless to say, there are not enough hours in a week to accommodate this number of patients at the Clinic, so approximately 95 per cent are treated by post. The results have gone beyond my wildest dreams. Our postal patients write to us or ring us if they have any worries regarding their treatment. They know we will do everything in our power to give them the correct advice and, when necessary, liaise with their GP on their behalf. The relationship between the Clinic and the medical profession gets better all the time, I am very happy to say; it is so satisfying when a doctor reports how pleased he or she is with the progress that a patient has made since beginning our treatment. Our patients also report to us how pleased their consultants and GPs are with their blood tests for things like erythrocyte sedimentation rate (ESR), C-reactive protein (CRP) and haemoglobin (Hb). Some of them are so well that the consultant does not want to see them again and they are discharged as fit after many years of useless, dangerous drug taking. I say 'useless' because the drugs given for arthritis *do not cure* and the unfortunate patient ends up with his or her arthritis and the side-effects of the drugs given for it. The side-effects can be very dangerous, even those of non-steroidal drugs. It is most disturbing to encounter from day to day the number of people with not just one or two life-threatening side-effects, but many. One patient writes:

> I have swallowed enough prescribed drugs to keep a small pharmacy in business for a year; drugs to stop the stiffness, drugs to stop the pain, drugs to attack the disease and drugs to stop the side-effects caused by the others. I have taken tablets every single day for over seven years, had numerous, painful injections into joints, plus frequent blood tests to check for side-effects – and *I've had enough*!

This is a typical story told by the majority of the first appointments seen at the Clinic, and what a sad story it is. Drugs are toxic in themselves, and, when given the patient is called upon to cope with the illness and the toxicity of the drug given for the illness. No heed is paid to the *cause* of the illness, and the drugs simply suppress the symptoms – *they cure nothing*.

There is continuous development and research into drugs, but yet again recent discoveries in drug therapy serve to emphasize my own belief that no drug is either safe or beneficial to the arthritis sufferer.

Understandably, people have great regard for their GPs and specialists, and find it daunting to consider questioning their advice.

This is where close contact with us at the Clinic can help a patient to find the right way forward gradually. Once people share their fears, anxieties and worries with us, we can advise them carefully on how to cope. Such patients become as friends, confiding those aspects of their lives that have such a great impact on their health. Such a rapport helps a person to recover – and most people seem to do just that.

When a patient defeats arthritis and regains full mobility and health, there is a terrific interest from family members and friends and from the patient's GP and consultant. We then have more people asking for help, not necessarily for arthritis, so gradually other conditions have required our research and attention. Life has become very busy indeed, but very early on in the life of the Clinic, my daughter Christine had come to help.

Towards the end of 1998, it gradually became apparent that my breathing was not so good, especially when I was worried or had exerted myself in some way. I visited the GP who instigated some tests at the hospital and discovered that my heart was the problem. When I was initially diagnosed at the age of 21 with rheumatoid arthritis, I had rheumatic fever and a badly enlarged heart. Although I recovered, I had a heart attack in my 40s and now the heart had decided to play up again. There was nothing to do except rest, so I found that I could not continue at my Clinic in Kenilworth; I had to give my heart a chance to recover once again.

Since 1981, Christine has been working alongside me, gradually developing her studies in Nutritional Medicine and gaining a firm understanding of the way in which I had been treating people with arthritis. I am so relieved that she is continuing the work that I started because there is such a thirst for knowledge among the people who contact us suffering with all kinds of arthritis, rheumatism, gout, polymyalgia rheumatica and so on. She has been able to continue where I have had to leave off and I am sure that arthritics will benefit enormously from her advice, care and attention. The Margaret Hills Clinic grew from my experiences and now Christine will continue with it, drawing upon her and her own family's health challenges to endorse and enhance our treatment for arthritis and allied diseases.

Postscript by Christine Horner – Margaret's daughter

Since this book was first published, my mother has given talks in a variety of venues to great crowds of people. They have been enjoyable to do and so rewarding. She has published several other books, some of which have been translated into other languages.

She has spoken on radio and television, and a film has been made and broadcast in the Middle East on the work of our Clinic. My mother retired around 1996; the enlarged heart slowed her down considerably. She had no arthritis, but her difficulties in walking and breathing had put a stop to her work at the Clinic, apart from occasionally writing an article for a newspaper or magazine. She saw a consultant heart specialist and was prescribed medication but didn't find it beneficial, so she stopped taking it. Gradually, she became housebound because of her heart condition.

It was at this time that I became aware of a Russian device that was supposed to be very helpful in treating heart problems. Intrigued, I arranged for Mum to be treated with the device as quickly as possible. Although it had only just been introduced into the UK and there was, as yet, little British evidence concerning its effectiveness, I'd been assured that it could be of great help and would have no ill effects.

We went to see a therapist called Penny who used the device. On arriving at Penny's home in Gloucestershire, we could see that it would take Mum a huge effort just to get inside the door. The driveway was uphill, so I parked the car as close as possible to the house. Next, we had to go up three steps to the front door, which, thankfully, had a handrail at the side. Mum hauled herself up, resting for a few minutes at each step, until finally she managed to get over the threshold and rest again. The treatment room was around the corner; the effort just to get there was overwhelming and, once more, Mum had to rest. After resting for 20 minutes or so, while I discovered more about the device, Mum managed to sit on the couch and then the treatment began. It was gentle, calm and soothing, and lasted about one hour. Understandably exhausted, Mum was thankful but relieved to start her journey home.

For two days following the treatment, Mum was more exhausted than ever and we were both very disappointed. I felt guilty for encouraging her to have the treatment but she was gracious in understanding what I was trying to do. No one in the UK had very much experience with this new device but we knew that it had been used to great effect for 20 years in Russia.

On the third day, though, everything changed. Mum woke up full of energy; she was excited and raring to go! Because we didn't know how long this improvement would last, Mum decided to take full advantage of it by going out into the fresh air, visiting the shops and enjoying the day. Well, the improvement did last; we gave Penny the good news and she promptly invited us for another session.

Penny was delighted to see Mum walk calmly up the steps this time! She gave her a second treatment that lasted about 45 minutes, and we made our way home. The following two days, Mum was back to square one: she was exhausted and had difficulty breathing, walking or talking. We were beginning to understand the pattern, though, for, on the third day, her energy soared. She cleaned her home throughout! This improvement continued for the rest of the week.

We went for a third session with Penny; it took about 30 minutes this time. Instead of the downturn we were expecting the following day, Mum continued to have good energy levels; she walked, talked and kept busy, and there were no adverse effects.

Despite Penny's inviting Mum for another session, she refused. She knew how much the sessions were taking me away from my clinic patients. She felt fine; she had great enthusiasm for the device and we determined that I should buy one and learn how to use it to the greatest effect.

What was this device that proved invaluable at such a stressful time? It was the self-controlled energo-neuro-adaptive regulation device or 'Scenar'. It triggers self-healing from the body's own immune system, setting up a dialogue between the brain and whichever part of the body requires healing.

From then on, with occasional treatments using my own Scenar device, Mum coped admirably until January 2003 but then her heart condition deteriorated more and more until she died peacefully in May 2003.

Her family – and all her patients who came to know her so well – will, of course, very sadly miss her. At the same time, we are very proud of all that she has achieved throughout her life. My mother had always attributed her knowledge, and successful results with her treatment, to God. It never ceased to amaze her that people showed such interest in her and cared so much for her. She felt that God had guided her throughout all aspects of her Clinic and developing her treatment to what it has become today.

I respect all that she has achieved and resist any attempts to change the treatment, regardless of up-and-coming research. I generally find the research confirms that the treatment outlined in this book is providing exactly what an arthritic needs – but in a relatively cheap, safe way, rather than by using expensive individual substances. The treatment that cured my mother has brought health and mobility back to thousands of people directly, or indirectly through the pages of this book. I keep up to date as much as possible and consider all new products coming on to the market to assess whether they will help our patients – after all, my mother used to say that she would have taken anything if she thought it would get rid of her pain. Arthritis sufferers are vulnerable to all new drugs and natural substances that might be of some help. I have added a new chapter in order to try and relate to the reader whether such substances could be useful to them. Such information is conveyed in the context of whether they would be a useful addition to the acid-free diet, acid-removing treatment of cider vinegar and honey drinks, molasses, Epsom salts baths, vitamins, minerals and protein that comprises the holistic healing programme devised by my mother.

I have worked alongside Margaret Hills since the early 1980s and it was her wish and my privilege that I should continue her work, ensuring that the appropriate advice, guidance and support are given. I have already been asked to speak on local radio, and have taken part in a 'phone-in' on arthritis, which was very successful, running on way past the allotted time – luckily on a Bank Holiday when the schedules were not so rigid! I will do my utmost to continue the work that my mother started so that more and more people can regain control of their health and start to live life to the full again!

Christine Horner, ECNP

Note on the fourth edition

I have added two appendices to the edition. The new Troubleshooting section should help determine what action to take if you feel you are not progressing as you expected. When individuals are trying to decide whether to undertake the Margaret Hills treatment, uppermost in their mind is 'what evidence do you have that it works?' This new edition brings an opportunity to incorporate the results of an initial study carried out under the auspices of the University of Hertfordshire. The study compared the effectiveness of treatment available for arthritis on the British NHS (National Health Service) with that from Margaret Hills.

Christine Horner, 2012

1

Arthritis – the cause and effects

According to the Arthritis and Rheumatism Council for Research, arthritis is Britain's most widespread disease. Before opening my Clinic, I spent six years as an Industrial Nurse, gaining first-hand experience of the suffering involved, and the sheer number of man-power days lost due to this awful disease. Surprisingly, the suffering is not confined to the middle-aged and elderly. Many children and teenagers suffer from arthritis, and more and more young people are taking cortisone and various other drugs prescribed for the condition. Basically, the term 'arthritis' describes the inflammation of a joint, or joints. The chief forms are osteoarthritis and rheumatoid arthritis, and the underlying cause of both is excess acidity in the body.

Acid is taken in over the years in the food we eat, and the liquids we drink. If our bodies contain the required nutrients to burn up the acid that we take in, then there is no problem. Unfortunately, the food we eat today is sadly lacking in those nutrients, so we are left with the situation of an undernourished body, full of acid. This acid is carried round in the blood, until it eventually deposits itself between the joints, on the bones, or in the muscles.

When acid is deposited in the muscles, we call the effect muscular rheumatism. Both arthritis and rheumatism are extremely painful conditions. If left alone they usually get worse, reducing the patient to a morbid state of existence, where there is excruciating pain with every movement. This was the state to which I was reduced when I was 36 years old. Looking back, I feel that it was all meant to be. I have yet to see a case of arthritis quite as bad as mine, but I now know that it was all brought about through years of unintentional 'wrong' eating and drinking.

I remember how I used to try to negotiate the stairs each evening, suffering unbearable pain. How I dreaded waking up each morning, manoeuvring my painful body several times before I managed to roll out of bed, crawling on all fours into a hot bath, in order to 'get started'. I can certainly sympathize with the patients at my Clinic, when they burst into tears with utter, hopeless depression.

When acids collect between joints, the pain on movement can be likened to a vicious stabbing. Sometimes the joints get locked and may stiffen altogether, until there is very little movement or, indeed, none at all. In some cases, the joints make a grating sound. This is called crepitus, the unpleasant sound of the joints moving on those hard acid deposits.

Every joint in the body is covered by a membrane which secretes synovial fluid, an oily substance which enables the joints to move freely, one on the other. When acid deposits form between the joints, a wearing away of that synovial membrane is very common, due to the continuous movement on those hard surfaces. Very often, there is also a wearing away of the actual surface of the joints themselves. When this occurs, it is a situation that cannot be reversed. However, with proper diet and treatment, the acid deposits can be dissolved away, alleviating the pain and halting the condition.

The vast majority of my patients, after six weeks of treatment, report considerably less pain and a general feeling of well-being that they have not experienced for years. This is mainly due to the nutritional supplements that are part of the treatment and, I feel, only goes to show that they had previously been existing in a very much undernourished body, full of toxic acid.

In 1928, at a conference in Bath, Sir W. Farquhar Buzzard (physician to King George V) was reported to have said that the medical profession did not know the cause of rheumatism – a disease that was costing the nation £20,000,000 every year, through loss of work. To date, not very much progress has been made. They now know the cause of rheumatism and arthritis, but do not know how to treat it effectively. Patients are pumped with drugs until their long-suffering, undernourished bodies can take no more. They are then told that there is no cure, and that they must 'learn to live with it'.

Nature cure practitioners everywhere recognize rheumatism as a disease caused by faulty diet. The same applies to arthritis, although this is a more serious disease, and will take longer to correct. The medical profession today is very seriously overworked and under-staffed. Doctors simply do not have the time to concentrate on each individual case, and unfortunately, the average person is largely unwilling to take the responsibility for his own health, while being quick to blame the doctor if he cannot produce an instant wonder-drug to put right the condition that has been unwittingly self-inflicted. The doctor is faced with a situation where there is a great deal of suffering borne through pain, very often hardship and frustration through loss of earning capacity, and worst of all, no hope for the future.

A girl of 18 came to my Clinic for consultation. She was an attractive girl, but her hands were deformed and she was in great pain. She told me that she was studying for her 'A' Levels, but when I asked her what she was hoping to do with her life, both she and her mother burst into tears. They told me that she had hoped to become a chemist, but since nothing could be done for her arthritis, she could not look forward to a career or marriage and, before long, would probably be confined to a wheelchair. What a sad, hopeless outlook for a young girl.

Day after day, the doctor is faced with this kind of situation, and since he has no effective 'tools' to work with, what a frustrating situation it must be for him. Doctors are very caring people – as a State Registered Nurse, I speak from experience. They have a tremendous responsibility to bear – that of their patients' health – and too often receive little gratitude for their efforts. Yet they persevere, still caring and mostly cheerful. If this book helps in any way to relieve the strain on doctors, and the suffering borne by arthritics, then it will have been well worth the effort involved.

Conditions related to arthritis

Rheumatism and arthritis are caused by excess acidity in the body. However, the reader may not be aware that these conditions are very often connected with cataracts, catarrh, hiatus hernia, diverticulitis, gallstones, kidney stones, and a host of other ailments, directly or indirectly related to faulty diet.

Refined sugar, white bread, refined cereals, beef and pork, are widely eaten today, and all leave behind them a residue of toxic acids in the body. Modern farming and refining techniques, and over-cooking or microwave cooking, destroy the alkaline mineral salts essential to the neutralization of these acids which, unchecked, soon pile up in the system. First to come under attack from the acids is the mucous membrane, a continuous sheath leading from mouth to anus. The primary build-up of acid in this area can cause those conditions previously mentioned. Eventually, the acid deposits itself between the joints, on the bones and in the muscles. We are then faced with a condition which can form the basis of many diseases in the body.

The body is now unable to function normally, and various pains occur – headaches, migraine, pains in the joints and muscles, cramps, pins and needles. The spine is very often the site of arthritis, resulting in severe misalignment of the vertebrae. Every area of the body is controlled by the nerves that run down the spinal column. Vertebrae fused by deposits of acid will invariably affect the part of the body that they serve. Let us take a look at the many areas of the body which may be affected by deposits of acid in the cervical, lumbar or dorsal vertebrae.

The cervical vertebrae

Deposits of acid in the cervical vertebrae may affect:

The blood supply to the head	The eyes/optic nerve	Neck muscles
The pituitary gland	Auditory nerve	Pharynx
The scalp	Sinuses	Neck glands
Bones of the face	Mastoid bones	Shoulders
The brain	Tongue, teeth, nose and lips	Tonsils
Inner and middle ear	Mouth and Eustachian tubes	Thyroid gland
Sympathetic nervous system	Vocal cords	Bursae in the shoulders and elbows

All this interference in the body may bring about:

headaches, nervousness, insomnia, head colds, high blood pressure, migraine, mental conditions, nervous breakdown, sleeping sickness, chronic neuralgia, tiredness, dizziness, vertigo, St Vitus's Dance, eye trouble, earache, fainting spells, neuritis,

acne, pimples, eczema, hay fever, catarrh, deafness, throat conditions, quinsy, stiff neck, pain in the upper arm, thyroid conditions
and certain cases of blindness.

The dorsal vertebrae

There are 12 dorsal vertebrae in the spinal column. Misalignment
here may cause functional heart conditions and chest pains. Also
at risk are the valves and coverings of the heart, the coronary
arteries, lungs, bronchial tubes, pleura and chest. Problems in these
areas can give rise to bronchitis, pleurisy, pneumonia, shortness of
breath, and pains in the lower arms and hands.

The gall bladder and common duct may be affected, leading to
gallstones, jaundice and shingles. The liver and solar plexus are
also dependent on this area of the spine for their healthy nerve
supply. Interference with the dorsal vertebrae may cause liver conditions to occur, plus anaemia, poor circulation, low blood pressure
and fevers. The stomach must also be included in this section,
impairment of which gives rise to indigestion, nervous stomach,
heartburn and dyspepsia. The pancreas, islets of Langerhans, and
the duodenum may be affected too, and interference with these
may result in diabetes, ulcers or gastritis.

Other parts of the body dependent on the proper alignment of
the dorsal vertebrae are:

Spleen	Kidneys	Fallopian tubes
Diaphragm	Urethra	Lymph glands
Adrenals	Small intestines	

Interference in these areas can cause:

hiccoughs, lowered resistance, allergies, hives, kidney trouble,
hardening of the arteries, chronic tiredness, nephritis, pyelitis,
skin conditions (such as acne, pimples, eczema or boils), and, in
certain circumstances, sterility.

All the aforementioned ailments may be directly attributed to
arthritis in the dorsal vertebrae.

Lumbar vertebrae

There are five lumbar vertebrae in the spinal column, and this is the area most commonly affected by misalignment due to arthritis. Arthritis in the lumbar region of the spine can give rise to:

constipation, colitis, dysentery, diarrhoea, ruptures, hernias, appendicitis, cramps, difficulty breathing, acidosis, varicose veins, bladder trouble, menstrual problems, bedwetting, impotence, menopause symptoms, and many knee pains.

Common complaints arising from arthritis in the lumbar vertebrae are:

sciatica, lumbago, painful or too frequent urination, and backache.

The lower legs, ankles and feet can also be affected by lumbar misalignment, resulting in:

Poor circulation in	Weak ankles and	Weakness in the
the legs	arches	legs
Swollen ankles	Cold feet	

The sacrum and coccyx may be affected, the former causing sacroiliac conditions and curvature of the spine, and the latter giving rise to haemorrhoids, pruritis, and pain at the end of the spine when sitting.

You will see from this long list of complaints that arthritis of the spine can set up in the body many continuous painful conditions, which make life unbearable for the long-suffering patient.

Of course, the spine is not the only place in the body subject to arthritis. It is very common in the hands, feet, shoulders and knees; in fact, any and every joint of the body is liable to come under attack from this disease. Arthritis attacks the bony structure of the body, and the reason for this is very simple to understand. Arthritis is caused by a build-up of acids in the body, mainly derived from years of faulty diet. When large quantities of acid steadily build up in the system, they have to deposit themselves somewhere, and unfortunately, they have a very great affinity with the bony structure of our bodies. This affinity is with the organic lime which is a prominent constituent of bony material.

Lime is an alkaline substance. By attraction of opposites, the acids in the body are inevitably drawn to this alkaline substance, for 'mutual neutralization'. The result of this process is an inflamed acid condition, which causes the joints to swell and become extremely tender and painful. Invariably, an affected joint feels stiff and becomes locked. Deformity then occurs, due to the erosive action on the bones of the acid impurities. The joint is now rendered incapable of performing its natural action. As a matter of interest, the lower parts of the body almost always seem to be the worst affected by chronic arthritis. I think this is because these lower parts bear the weight of the body. Also, the blood circulation is not as active in the lower regions. Acid deposits will also be attracted to wherever there has been an operation or previous injury, or any area of the body put under undue stress.

Gout is a condition very often associated with arthritis. Gout was once considered to be a rich man's disease – due to the theory that it was caused by excessive alcohol consumption. Here again, the culprit is a surfeit of acid waste in the blood and tissues, no doubt aggravated by years of poor diet. I have often been asked if arthritis and gout are hereditary – well, of course, they can be. If an expectant mother's body is full of acid, there is a great possibility that her baby will be born with too much acid in the blood. This may give rise, very early in childhood, to digestive disorders, a tendency to colds and catarrh, bronchial troubles and, very often, infantile eczema and other skin disorders.

I have recently been alarmed by the increasing number of child sufferers from arthritis. A child is entirely dependent on its mother for a healthy start in life. If the mother is not educated as to the necessary kind of nourishing foods to eat, in order to maintain her own bodily health, there is very little hope that the developing foetus will obtain the healthy start that is its right. There is a saying: 'The hand that rocks the cradle rules the world' – how true! The health of the nation is dependent upon mothers. Without a healthy nation, we cannot expect the output of our workforce to be of the quality necessary to maintain a first-class economy.

A little girl aged 11 arrived at the Clinic; she was tired and depressed. She had been in ill health since birth and was diagnosed with chronic juvenile arthritis at the age of eight. She also had lichen sclerosis. She was in tremendous pain – her hips, knees, ankles, back and neck caused her the most discomfort. She was taking antibiotics, non-steroidal anti-inflammatory drugs (NSAIDs) and paracetamol, and also applying steroid cream. Her consultant had provided an active treatment plan of exercises and swimming, along with splints and a wheelchair. I worked out a programme for her and, after persevering for three months, she was able to report that she had had no pain whatsoever for four consecutive weeks. She persisted with the programme, but two months later her knees locked; she was confined to her wheelchair, and admitted to hospital. She and her parents refused medications and, within four to five days, her legs were back to normal and she was discharged with the note that she had 'never had arthritis'. She had no sign of arthritis in her blood or on X-rays; no aches or swellings; and was back doing PE and running a mile!

The little girl's body was in a much healthier state; she had learned what she needed to eat and drink – and what to avoid – and so too had her parents. So the whole family benefited and the future was much brighter for them.

People are generally unaware of their body's requirements, or of what nutrition is needed in order to maintain bodily health. Ironically, those with the most money seem to be those most likely to exist in a vitamin-deficient diet, often over-indulging in alcohol. One does not need to be rich to eat for health. Fresh vegetables and fruit, for example, are still relatively cheap and easy to obtain, as are cheese, chicken and fish, which provide sufficient protein for a healthy diet. Later in this book, I shall be talking in more detail about the diets necessary to arthritis-free living, with regard to both prevention and cure.

Patients often tell me that their arthritis began when they fell, broke a limb, pulled a muscle, or strained a tendon. They therefore attribute their arthritis to the injury. However, this is not directly the case, although to a person uninitiated into the cause of arthritis, it certainly may appear to be so.

When an injury occurs to any part of the body, an alkaline reaction is set up at the site of that injury. As I have already mentioned, the acids in the body are inevitably attracted to this alkaline site for mutual neutralization. The resulting effect is a 'triggering off' of a rheumatic condition, causing both pain and swelling in the affected area. If a joint is involved, decalcification may occur in the bones, giving rise to deformity and loss of power and movement. However, if a person does not have too much uric acid in the system to begin with, this situation will not arise. The natural healing power of the body will immediately come to the rescue, thereby promoting the health of the limb concerned without further complications. The reader may deduce from the foregoing statement that the cause of arthritis at the site of an injury is not due to the injury itself, but rather to the toxic state of the whole body.

The food and drink we partake of are overwhelmingly important. This cannot be over-stressed. In addition, the lifestyle can contribute to a build-up of acid. Overwork, 'burning the candle at both ends', insufficient restful sleep, medications of all kinds (including antibiotics, vaccinations and so-called recreational drugs), emotional and relationship difficulties such as those concerned with divorce and with the balancing of childcare and work, are all relatively new issues that assail us in this day and age. Some people try to do too much and to cram so much into each day that their health is bound to take a downward turn as the stress takes its toll. The result is often some form of arthritis, fibromyalgia, polymyalgia rheumatica, rheumatism – sometimes mild aches and pains, at other times devastating, traumatic, excruciating, all-consuming pain.

I am often asked if there is such a thing as 'spontaneous remission', that is, when the disease disappears for no obvious reason. I must say that I do not think there is. What may seem a natural remission to the uninitiated is, in reality, the body's own healing powers overcoming the disease, but it is my opinion that no disease will just bow out gracefully, adopting the attitude of 'OK, you win', without a determined effort of self-help being undertaken by the sufferer.

From the foregoing chapter, it should be very obvious to the reader why no 'magic drug' has yet been found to cure or relieve arthritis. In the following chapter I shall describe the drugs which are currently available, their dangerous side-effects, and their inefficiency in the treatment and cure of arthritis.

2

Drugs and their side-effects

Arthritis is systemic – meaning that once it appears in any one joint there is no doubt that there are deposits of toxic acid throughout the patient's entire body. Perhaps these deposits have not, as yet, become inflamed, but sooner or later they will, reducing the sufferer to a debilitating and excruciatingly painful state of immobility. As I have said before, there is no magic drug that will give lasting relief from arthritis, simply because the patient's body is loaded with acid deposits, which must be got rid of before one can hope for any long-term success.

At present, arthritis is treated either with drugs, painkillers or surgery. When a joint becomes inflamed, the doctor will usually prescribe an anti-inflammatory drug which, as a rule, will suppress the inflammation, halt the condition, and thus bring relief – but only temporarily. Before long, the inflammation will rear its ugly head again, causing more pain than ever. A stronger and more powerful drug will then be administered, and the story repeats itself until invariably the joint or joints concerned become so tender and stiff that the slightest movement brings intense pain. The patient eventually becomes immune to the drugs administered and the only course left open to the frustrated doctor is to suggest a new hip joint, knee joints or whatever.

The unfortunate patient is then directed to the Rheumatologist who will put him on the waiting list. Many of my patients have been on the waiting list for at least two years for an operation of this kind. While on the waiting list, they are pumped with anti-rheumatic drugs which set up day by day side-effects in their bodies, that invariably lead to some form of 'doctor-induced' disease. Hospitals today are full of patients who have fallen victim to the side-effects of drugs and antibiotics. Drugs drain the body of nutrition, especially iron, and the vast majority of patients on drugs are anaemic. Many are aware of the dangers of such treatment and are very loath to accept any form of drug. Unfortunately, when pain becomes intense – as it does with arthritis – the sufferer feels such a burden to himself, and to others, that he has no alternative but to submit to a course of treatment which may, but very often does not, relieve his suffering.

Of course, a new joint will not remove the acids that are causing the trouble. Sooner or later, another hip or knee joint, or perhaps both, will be necessary. The saga starts all over again until eventually the long-suffering patient is reduced to a state of depression and hopelessness.

According to *Baillière's Nurses' Dictionary*, the word 'drug' means 'any substance used as a medicine' and if we think of them in that light then of course there is no getting away from the fact that they are very useful substances indeed; and have a definite place in medicine today. When drugs are taken repeatedly, a lot of patients become dependent on them and are unable to do without them either emotionally or physically. Then this is called drug addiction and the majority of people today are well aware of the sad state of helplessness that is the result of such dependence.

Most patients that attend my Clinic do so with a burning desire to be able to function without their drugs. They have come to realize how dependent on them they are becoming and they also realize that the prolonged consumption of them is having very undesirable side-effects.

One of the most common treatments for arthritis – aspirin – was introduced in 1899. Aspirin is a derivative of salicylic acid and although it is considered one of the least toxic of the drugs it can be dangerous to some people. Every person's make-up is different and the human body is a very complex machine. 'One man's meat is another man's poison' and what suits one person may be very damaging to another. Fortunately, I was able to tolerate the 12 aspirins a day that I was taking without experiencing any side-effects but to another that dosage, or even much less, could cause vomiting, headaches or high temperature. Aspirin can also give rise to deafness and noises in the ear and it is widely known that this drug can cause bleeding of the stomach, possibly even resulting in ulceration. This in turn can lead to anaemia due to the constant blood loss. In fact, aspirin can cause severe irritation of the whole alimentary tract from stomach to anus. Paracetamol is now favoured for these reasons and is often prescribed initally alongside physiotherapy and occupational therapy.

Various drugs are used in the primary treatment of arthritis – these include ibuprofen, diclofenac, celecoxib, naproxen and so on. Some patients report to me that from the time they started to take some of these drugs they felt ill with various symptoms such as headache, nausea, vomiting, unpleasant noises in the ears, etc. Others say these drugs gave a lot of relief to begin with but very soon the pain became so bad that they were prescribed stronger drugs, such as methotrexate, sulfasalazine, penicillamine, steroids and steroid injections – among a lot of others. Drugs to protect the stomach are routinely prescribed alongside them.

In June 2011, research from the Medical Research Council Cognitive Function and Ageing Studies project showed that a side-effect of many commonly used drugs is an increase in the risk of both cognitive brain impairment, such as dementia, and death in older people. This study from the University of East Anglia, which involved more than 13,000 people aged over 65, was the first systematic investigation into the long-term health impacts of many prescription and over-the-counter drugs.

The medicines that can affect brain function negatively are wide-ranging and many are frequently taken by older people; the more drugs taken for multiple health problems, the greater the likelihood that the individual will be affected.

Co-author Professor Carol Brayne, principal investigator of the project at the University of Cambridge, stressed the importance of scrutinizing very carefully medications given to older people to minimize the risks of brain dysfunction and death. Dr Chris Fox, Clinical Senior Lecturer at Norwich Medical School, advised that regular review of their medications – both prescribed and over-the-counter – should be carried out, and that prescribing multiple drugs should be avoided. As the elderly are more commonly afflicted by arthritis, and the majority of them are on drugs of one form or another then, of course, the foregoing comments apply in large measure. In my opinion, some drugs made for the treatment of arthritis are among the most dangerous drugs made, and when taken over a long period of time they can create the most undesirable side-effects, as evidenced by the following studies.

Increased risk of skin cancer

In August 2011, Deborah Symmons, Professor of Rheumatology and Musculoskeletal Epidemiology at Arthritis Research UK Epidemiology Unit, said: 'We have known for some time that there may be a slightly increased risk of skin cancer in patients using anti-TNF drugs' (*Annals of the Rheumatic Diseases*, 70 (11), pp. 1895–1904). Anti-TNF drugs, such as abatacept, etanercept, infliximab, adalimumab, certolizumab, golimumab, rituximab, anakinra and tocilizumab, are sometimes prescribed to block the action of a protein called TNF (tumour necrosis factor) and thereby reduce inflammation. These drugs are also known as cytokine modulators or biologics and are used for rheumatoid arthritis.

Increased risk of contracting *Clostridium difficile* (C. diff.) infection

When non-steroidal anti-inflammatory drugs (NSAIDs, e.g. ibuprofen, naproxen and diclofenac) and Cox-2 inhibitor drugs (e.g. celecoxib and etoricoxib) are prescribed, it is acknowledged that they can adversely affect the digestive and gastrointestinal tract, so a 'stomach protector' is also often given – 'stomach protectors' are proton pump inhibitors, such as lansoprazole and omeprazole. They are also used to treat heartburn and acid reflux. However, in October 2010 a series of studies in the Archives of Internal Medicine suggested that the overuse of proton pump inhibitors increased the risk of patients 'contracting an intestinal infection caused by *Clostridium difficile* bacteria'.

Increased risk of weaker bones and fractures

The same study commented that overuse of proton pump inhibitors 'may increase the risk of fractures . . . These medicines work by reducing the acid in the stomach which may make it difficult for the body to absorb the calcium that is necessary for healthy bones.'

Increased risk of heart attack and stroke

In a section on Cox-2 inhibitors, the Medicines and Healthcare products Regulatory Agency (MHRA) raises concerns about cardiovascular safety:

Whilst Cox-2 selective anti-inflammatory medicines may be useful for some patients, recent evidence indicates that patients treated with selective Cox-2 inhibitors may be at a slightly increased risk of cardiovascular problems such as heart attacks and strokes. Rofecoxib (Vioxx and Vioxx Acute) was withdrawn in September 2004 because of evidence of increased risk after long-term treatment.

With regard to safety, the best drug is considered to be ibuprofen, but combining any NSAID with aspirin heightens the risk of gastro-intestinal side-effects.

To illustrate how dangerous these medications can be, possible side-effects include:

hypersensitivity reactions, headache, dizziness, nervousness, depression, drowsiness, insomnia, vertigo, hearing disturbances such as tinnitus, photosensitivity and haematuria. Blood disorders and fluid retention may occur. NSAIDs should be used with caution in the elderly and in allergic disorders. Long-term use of some NSAIDS may be connected with reduced female fertility. Most manufacturers advise avoiding the use of NSAIDs during pregnancy and during breast-feeding if possible.

It just goes to show that the safest drug is certainly not *safe*.

In February 1991, the *British Journal of Rheumatology* published the following report:

Treating tennis elbow with steroid injections is totally useless, a study has concluded. Rheumatologists at Guy's Hospital, London, compared hydrocortisone, triamcionlone and lignocaine injections in 88 patients. The doctors measured pain, tenderness and grip over 24 weeks and discovered that steroid injections 'were probably of transient benefit and did not influence a trend towards healing'. The jabs also caused bad side-effects.

When disease-modifying anti-rheumatic drugs (DMARDs) such as methotrexate, azathioprine, hydroxychloroquine, ciclosporin, leflunomide and sulfasalazine are prescribed for rheumatoid arthritis, psoriatic arthritis or juvenile arthritis, regular full blood counts, and renal and liver function tests are required because the drugs can have serious effects; most are contraindicated in pregnancy and breastfeeding. Eye testing is recommended, as ocular toxicity can occur.

Anti-TNF medications (e.g. infliximab and etanercept) pre-scribed for severe active rheumatoid arthritis are associated with an increased risk of infection, which can become severe; other side-effects include those typical with NSAIDs. Orthodox medical treatment remains potentially dangerous, and arthritis drugs are prone to many side-effects, which may affect an individual patient.

When the arthritis sufferer becomes aware that the drug pre-scribed is not actually making him or her feel very much better, another drug is added. It is common now to find that combinations of drugs are prescribed with the hope of preventing progression of the disease. The combination of drugs prescribed to a patient may still not 'control' the disease, and yet the possibility of side-effects is great. The drugs add to the toxic load in the body and the general health can deteriorate as a result.

In contrast to the above reports, an October 1991 study, pub-lished in the medical journal *The Lancet* and entitled 'Controlled trial of fasting and one-year vegetarian diet in rheumatoid arthritis', showed that in some patients, a substantial reduction in the symp-toms of rheumatoid arthritis could be obtained by fasting followed by an individually adjusted vegetarian diet. Although fasting had previously been found to be an effective treatment for the condi-tion, most patients deteriorated when they started eating again.

In the study, 27 patients were admitted to a Norwegian health farm for four weeks and allowed only herbal tea, garlic, vegetable broths and juices for the first seven to ten days. They were given meat-free and gluten-free food to eat every second day. Any food that caused joint pain and stiffness on two separate occasions was withdrawn.

Dairy products, fish, citrus fruit, salt, refined sugar, strong spices, tea, coffee and alcohol were banned for the first three and a half months. After this period, milk and other dairy products and food containing gluten were reintroduced one at a time into the diet. The researchers at the National Hospital, Oslo, reported that after the first month patients showed a significant improvement in the number of tender and swollen joints, that they were in less pain and had stronger hand grips. They went on to say:

> Despite the difficulties of covering essential nutritional needs during the first four months we do not believe this diet carries a

health risk. On the contrary, it seems to be a useful supplement to the ordinary medical treatment of rheumatoid arthritis.

The researchers suggested that a switch to a vegetarian diet caused major changes in dietary fatty acids which they believed might reduce inflammatory activity in arthritis.

This report is encouraging and shows that doctors are at last investigating diet and nutrition in relation to arthritis. However, in my opinion, instead of drawing the conclusion that a vegetarian diet could be a useful supplement to medical treatment, they should be thinking of it in the place of medical treatment, that is, drugs and their accompanying side-effects.

There is a huge cost involved in the medical treatment of someone with arthritis, which incorporates not only drugs but also GPs, nurses, specialist physicians and surgeons, physiotherapists, occupational therapists, social workers and so on – quite apart from the enormous indirect costs related to loss of the ability to work. It stands to reason that personal responsibility in diet and lifestyle ought to be taken by all arthritis sufferers if there is even the slightest chance that such measures could be beneficial. In fact, the measures outlined in this book can make a terrific difference.

Doctors are well aware of the side-effects of the drugs they prescribe, but can do little about it. Invariably, the person is unwilling to help him- or herself. Drugs are far too easily obtained. The line of least resistance is often preferred to a project of self-help which merely involves a little effort and planning a correct diet.

Prevention is far better than cure and I feel I must emphasize how invaluable a good nutritional education would be to both boys and girls during their last years at school. The majority have little, if any, idea of how to look after their bodies by eating the correct foods necessary for healthy living. After all, the body is the second most special possession we have in this world – the soul being the first.

In the following chapter, I will tell you how to remove the toxic acids from the body that are causing your arthritis and enlarge upon the reasons for adopting the 'natural' method of treatment.

3

The treatment of arthritis
by natural means

Arthritis is mainly a disease of dietetic origin. By recognizing this, and treating it accordingly, I have had the most remarkable and gratifying results. I was able to rescue myself from a state of hopeless incapacity and pain, to achieve an excellent state of health, that I had not known for years. I was able to raise eight children, foster another, and eventually take a refresher course in nursing. Although I had been away from nursing for 30 years, I found that I had both the strength and the mental ability to 'pick up the threads' and renew my career. Following my recovery, I continued to work full-time as an Industrial Nurse, until two years ago, when I decided to set up a clinic for arthritics at my home in Coventry. The results that I have experienced since opening the Clinic have been most encouraging and have far exceeded my expectations.

We have established that arthritis is caused by excess acidity in the body, and that this imbalance is created by a lack of the required nutrients necessary to the neutralization of the acid we absorb from our daily diet and create with our lifestyle. The quality of food available today often leaves much to be desired. Many of the nutrients which should be supplied in our food are destroyed by the addition of chemicals and pesticides. To the farmer, a greater yield is the most important factor, but such additions result in a sacrifice of quality and the supply of organically grown fruit and vegetables is extremely limited. This limitation makes it very necessary for us to take food supplementation, in the form of vitamins, minerals and proteins. This applies not only to arthritics, but also to the very young, schoolchildren, adolescents, expectant mothers, nursing mothers, sports and business people, and of course, the elderly. Having firmly established the cause of arthritis, let us now turn our thoughts to the successful treatment and elimination of this disease.

I believe that there is only one sensible way to relieve, and possibly cure, arthritis:

1 The patient must adopt a method of treatment that will eliminate toxic acids from the body.
2 The patient must adhere to an acid-free diet, in order to prevent any further intake of acid.
3 The patient must restore nutrients necessary to the 'burning up' of acids in the body.

In the following pages, I will detail, and explain, the regime that I adopted, after extensive research into the natural treatment of arthritis. Having been trained in conventional medicine, based on treatments by drugs such as antibiotics, it was with rather a negative attitude that I approached the 'natural cure' method. However, I knew that I had nothing to lose by it and thought that even if it did me no good, at least it could do me no harm.

Before starting the treatment, I discarded the splints from my painful, swollen hands, and threw away the collar that was gradually locking my neck. I took off my surgical corset, and removed the built-up arches from my shoes. I was then ready to work on removing the excess acid, and all signs of arthritis, from my body.

First, and most important of all, I developed a positive attitude. Remember, good health must be earned. In your fight for health, keep cheerful and optimistic. The correct mental attitude is a fundamental necessity if you are to have any chance of success. In disease of any nature, the nervous system suffers traumatically and a direct result of this is depression, fear and anxiety. When one develops a hopeful, optimistic and forward-looking attitude, one paves the way for greater success. Think the following: 'Disease has no part in my life, and I am going to get better.' So thinking, I faced each day with renewed energy. I pictured myself full of radiant health and vitality and convinced myself that each day brought me one step nearer to my goal.

Having developed a positive frame of mind, I turned my attention to the removal of the toxic acids from my body. The 'prescription' that I adopted was as follows:

1 On rising, I dissolved one teaspoon of clear honey in a tumbler of hot water, and added to this one dessertspoon of cider vinegar. I took this mixture three times a day.
2 I took one teaspoon of black molasses three times daily.
3 I took an Epsom salts bath three times per week.
4 I took a full range of the best quality vitamins, minerals and proteins each day, in order to replace in my body the nutrition that had become so depleted. This was also to help in the burning up of the acids that had invaded my body and caused such havoc. These vitamins, minerals and protein are now made for me especially for my arthritic patients and are available from the Clinic. We call them the 'Margaret Hills Formula and Protein'.
5 I exercised my joints gently. Every book that I had read advocated the benefits of walking in the fresh air. However, I could not walk, so I had to make do with gentle, indoor exercise, but I always ensured that my room was well ventilated.

I hoped that this regime would remove those toxic acids that were causing my trouble. I was, nevertheless, amazed when after only two weeks on this treatment, I definitely began to feel better. I had more strength, suffered less depression, and was certainly sleeping more easily.

A month went by, and the ease with which I moved my fingers became more noticeable. Of course, I had my bad days, but I was not worried. The natural cure books had told me to expect this, as it results from the body's attempt to 'throw off' the acids. From time to time, while following the treatment, the patient may find that his joints become inflamed and painful. This does not last for very long, and when one knows what to expect it is so much easier to weather the storm. I consoled myself with the thought that tomorrow I would feel better, and that gradually the pain would go away, never to return. A hopeful attitude does much more to alleviate pain than does any drug. Each week brought fresh improvement and the joy in my heart when I managed to walk from the lounge to the kitchen was immeasurable. I knew then that I was getting better. The improvement quickened, so I persevered with the treatment. By the end of 12 months, I had changed from being nervous, irritable, and depressed to being a calm, joyful, agile and healthy person. I was ready, and willing, to resume my place as a wife and mother, full of renewed strength and vigour and more anxious to please and care for my family than ever before. I was so grateful to the Lord for giving me the strength and encouragement to explore all avenues, in an effort to help myself.

I have kept myself very busy through the ensuing years, and as a result have made many social contacts. I have tried never to miss an opportunity to spread the news to suffering arthritics, many of whom have since had amazing results with this natural method of treatment. I have found that it always pays dividends to explain to my patients why they should do what I ask them to. It usually takes about one-and-a-half hours to explain in detail the reasons why they should take cider vinegar, honey and molasses, and the benefits to be gained from Epsom salts baths. I also explain the necessity of an acid-free diet, and describe which foods to avoid. Last, I explain the very important part played in the treatment by the wholefood nutrition that I prescribe.

The components of a natural cure

Cider vinegar

This excellent product is made from mature cider apples and is a combination of minerals, organic matter and acetic acid. In order to be fit, we must have enough sleep and exercise and, of course, a well-balanced diet. A regular intake of cider vinegar can help keep one free of arthritis. I think this is largely due to the fact that cider vinegar regulates the body's metabolism, through the quantities of minerals that it contains.

The hard acid deposits connected with arthritis are very similar in substance to the shell of an egg. Cider vinegar has the power to dissolve those acid deposits so they pass out naturally, via the kidneys. The reader can carry out an experiment to show how this works. Place an egg, complete with shell, in a jar or glass. Cover the egg with 'neat' cider vinegar and in two days the shell will have completely dissolved, leaving the egg intact. Similarly, when cider vinegar saturates the bloodstream, it gets between the joints, dissolving the acid deposits and passing them away. Cider vinegar contains malic acid. This should not be confused with the harmful acids which have collected between the joints, on the bones, or in the muscles, causing arthritis.

One has to remember that the longer one has had arthritis, the longer it will be before any noticeable results are obtained. I suffered from arthritis for 16 years, and after one month on the treatment, could see only a slight improvement. I could so easily have given up, but knew that if this treatment did not work I had very little hope of achieving any cure at all. I persevered, and within 12 months had rid myself of every sign of arthritis.

Arthritics are often overweight, due to the inactivity forced upon them. Their joints are so painful on movement that the natural reaction is to minimize the pain by keeping still. Arthritics also tend to eat convenience foods, which require little effort in their preparation. Thus they survive on a diet high in calories and low in nutrients, which only adds to their weight problem, making them less and less mobile. Cider vinegar is a natural diuretic, and thus acts to some extent as a slimming agent in overweight people. Most of my patients return after six weeks, absolutely thrilled because they have managed to lose weight without any effort. As a result, they feel better in themselves, and this gives them fresh hope for the future.

As I have said, for the first few weeks on the treatment, patients may experience pain in places they have not known it before. The pain is not stronger than before, but rather than being confined to the joints already involved, it now appears to be all over the body. If one gives this a little thought, one can understand the reason why. The patient's blood has been saturated with cider vinegar, which has set to work on all those acid deposits, churning them up, and dissolving them away. This process will inevitably cause some pain and the patient may be forgiven for thinking that the treatment is doing more harm than good. Unfortunately, some patients are tempted to give up at this early stage, thereby losing the value of the treatment, just as it has begun to take effect. This is, indeed, a pity. When the sufferer experiences this reaction, he should think: 'It is the treatment working for me; in a week or two, the pain will pass and I will get better.'

When a patient has been affected with arthritis for some considerable time, continuous movement of the joints on those hard acid deposits often causes a wearing away of the actual surface of the joints. This is a situation that cannot be reversed, but it is possible to halt the condition and lessen the pain. This in itself is well worth striving for.

'Wear and tear' is a very general term used by the medical profession, as is 'crumbling of the joints', and 'premature ageing of the bones'. I have found that most patients who come to my clinic attach tremendous importance to each word that falls from the doctor's lips and as a result often take on an attitude of hopelessness that is not easy to overcome. 'You have arthritis, and must learn to live with it' is a very common statement in the doctor's surgery. In the majority of cases, when a patient asks his doctor if this condition has anything to do with diet, the reply is usually 'no'. I do appreciate the strain that doctors are under, but I believe that the condition has everything to do with diet, and can be simply treated with an acid-free diet. After all, 'you are what you eat'. If a plant receives the wrong food, it will wither and die. As with other living things, our whole well-being hinges on diet.

Many arthritics also suffer from high blood pressure, angina, or some form of circulatory disease. The taking of cider vinegar can be most beneficial in this case, as it is known to be a 'blood normalizer'. If the blood pressure is too high, cider vinegar will help bring it down to normal, and if too low, it will raise it accordingly.

Ridges sometimes appear on the nails, due to lack of calcium salts in the tissues. This deficiency can also affect the bones, teeth and hair. Cider vinegar can help this condition enormously, as it encourages the body to make more effective use of the calcium derived from food. Among other things, a lack of calcium in the tissues will result in thin and brittle nails, dull hair, tooth decay and brittle bones. Cramps and pins and needles are also closely associated with calcium deficiency. Cider vinegar, by assisting in the absorption of calcium, can play a large part in the correction of these abnormalities.

It should be noted that you can expect to urinate more frequently while taking cider vinegar, due to the diuretic effect it has on the body. For the reader who does not suffer from arthritis but would like to avoid it, two teaspoons of well-diluted cider vinegar taken three times daily will, I believe, act as a preventive measure.

It should now be clear to the reader that cider vinegar is a very valuable commodity in the treatment of arthritis. After six weeks of taking cider vinegar, people usually report a transformation in their skin, hair and nails, leading their friends to ask what is it they are doing, as they are looking so much better. The benefits of taking cider vinegar are endless, but I hope that I have sufficiently evaluated its use in the relief of arthritis and associated ailments. As a point of interest, I highly recommend the use of unfiltered organic apple cider vinegar which still retains the 'mother'.

Honey

Honey – as we all know – comes from bees, and is produced to a larger or smaller degree in every country in the world. The two predominant types of sugar present in honey are fructose and glucose. These sugars are 'pre-digested' and can be used immediately by the body, to produce 'instant energy'. When ordinary sugar is taken into the body, it cannot be used immediately, due to the delay while digestive processes act.

Honey is packed with natural vitamins, minerals and trace elements. Among other, lesser ingredients, honey contains:

proteins	magnesium	phosphorus
calcium	selenium	pollen
copper	acids and amino acids	sodium
silica	chlorine	manganese
iron	potassium	nitrogen
lime	sulphur	

The composition of honey is affected by the types of flowers and plants from which the nectar is collected and also by the nature of the soil wherein the plants grow. The time of year and prevailing weather conditions at time of collection can also affect its composition. The type of flower or plant from which the nectar is taken also greatly influences the flavour of honey and its colour.

Darker honeys contain much more iron than light-coloured honey. I have found, in treating arthritics, that the vast majority are suffering from acute iron deficiency. Many have been taking drugs which have drained the body of iron. Lack of iron in the body can lead to all kinds of blood disorders, anaemia especially. This makes the patient feel tired and listless; a marked dullness of the eyes and lifeless hair are very common signs. As the patient feels 'drained', the most sensible course of action is to introduce a good, organic source of iron to promote instant energy. Honey is such a source.

Most of the 'B complex' range of vitamins can be found in honey, and it is these that feed the nerves. Most arthritics are in a highly nervous state. They feel pain very acutely, have sleepless nights, and become very depressed. The depression is caused first by the stress of the complaint, and second by the utter hopelessness the patients feel, when told that they must 'learn to live with it'. Honey is a most beneficial food for the tired, nervous and highly strung arthritis sufferer. Most arthritics, especially the advanced cases, have sleepless nights when they are racked with pain. Many pace the floor for hours during the night, suffering either from cramp or pins and needles or both. Patients have told me that they wake in the morning wishing they did not have to live through another day. This attitude of mind also brings great stress to the patient's family.

As a rule, if the patient is not overweight, I recommend the taking of honey in large amounts, usually one dessertspoon to be taken three times daily. Very often, during the first week of treatment, patients experience a sense of calm that they have not known for years. This, in itself, is wonderful, and patients settle down to their prescribed regime full of hope for a future with less, or even no pain.

Obviously some patients take longer than others to show signs of improvement, but I have never yet heard it said that the treatment has not done any good.

Honeys containing a lot of pollen are very rich in vitamin C. This is an extremely important vitamin that we need daily but, unfortunately, it cannot be stored by the body. As a rule, we depend on fruit and vegetables for our vitamin C intake, but owing to its instability, this vitamin can be easily lost or reduced during preparation and cooking. For example, freshly squeezed orange juice, left in the refrigerator for a few days, will have lost a significant amount of its vitamin C content. It is hard to know how much vitamin C we are getting from our food. Stress and smoking – a habit associated with stress – may affect our body's need for this vitamin. What better source to derive it from, than natural, pure honey?

As a point of interest, I have found honey to be very effective in the healing of ulcers and burns. Many hospitals today are reverting to the use of honey in these cases, as it is a natural antibiotic, and I have yet to find anyone who is allergic to it.

Black molasses

Molasses is made from raw, unsulphured cane sugar. It is a black, treacle-like substance, packed with nutrients, and may be taken at any time when most convenient. I usually recommend a dose of one teaspoonful to be taken three times daily. Molasses can be taken undiluted, but if so, should be followed immediately by a drink of warm water as it has a tendency to discolour the teeth. I found one teaspoon of molasses dissolved in four ounces of warm water to be right for me. Taken like this, it is easily assimilated, more digestible, and it will not stain the teeth. Those with delicate stomachs, who may find that a teaspoonful is too much at one time, may take it in smaller, more frequent doses. If preferred, molasses can be taken on toast – wholemeal of course! There is very little nutrition in white bread, as the husk and kernel of the wheat have been extracted, leaving it deficient in fibre, vitamins and minerals.

Molasses may also be taken on porridge, or mixed with marmalade. However it is taken, as a food packed with iron and minerals, molasses is a wonderful blood-cleanser for arthritics. Like honey, molasses is also a marvellous external and internal healer. As I have said, arthritics are prone to suffer from stomach ulcers, diverticulitis and similar conditions, caused by the acids eating away at the stomach and colon walls. As a rule, after taking molasses for one week, my patients report that these ailments are giving them less trouble. For external growths, boils, sores and cuts, molasses mixed with a little water and applied as a poultice is a wonderful, natural ointment. Molasses is also a laxative. Most people can take two teaspoons per day without experiencing any undue relaxation of the bowels, but as each case differs, I usually leave it to the individual to regulate his own intake. Used as a laxative, however, I always advise the patient to start with one teaspoonful per day, increasing the dosage, as the body becomes accustomed to it.

Like honey, molasses is a rich source of iron and can alleviate that tired feeling from which so many suffer. It is also a rich source of

B vitamins, and so feeds the nerves, relieving spells of deep depression, bouts of painful neuralgia, and debilitating attacks of colds and influenza. Molasses also contains copper and magnesium, and is extremely high in pantothenic acid and inositol. Crude, raw sugar cane molasses contains about 50 per cent fruit sugar, and can be used as a substitute for sugar on cereals and puddings, stirred into milk, or eaten in place of jam or jelly.

Molasses also contains a large amount of phosphoric acid and potassium. A combined deficiency of these in the body causes a breakdown of the cells, especially those of the brain and nerves. Anxiety uses up potassium salts in the blood and tissues and can produce a relapse in the treatment of arthritis. Here again, the taking of sugar cane molasses can be of great benefit, as it is very rich in potassium salts.

As I have mentioned before, excess acidity in the body may give rise to gastric ulcers. The majority of medical practitioners realize that ulcers do not occur unless there is a deficiency of certain mineral salts in the tissues. Molasses replaces those mineral salts in the blood and tissues, thereby promoting a healing of the ulcers, wherever they may be. Many patients suffer from external ulcers, due to an attempt by the body to rid itself of toxic acids. Little can be gained from merely treating the local condition – a 'whole person' regime must be adopted. Thorough 'dietary cleansing' will remove the excess acid from the body, although a localized poultice of molasses and water may also be applied to good effect.

Many forms of skin disease are connected with arthritis, for example, eczema, dermatitis, psoriasis. 'Suppressive' ointments, firm favourites with the doctors, do much more harm than they do good. When applied to skin rashes and ulcers, they suppress the infection, driving it further into the body only to set up a more serious complaint elsewhere. Treatment of the 'whole person', through internal cleansing with molasses, can be of great help in dealing with these conditions, and external poultices of molasses will speed up the healing process.

High blood pressure, angina and weak hearts are very often associated with arthritis. These diseases have been known to respond extremely well to the 'molasses treatment'. Constipation and colitis are yet other conditions often connected with arthritis, and in these instances patients are normally advised to adopt a high-fibre diet. However, this is only half the story. Very often, a loss of muscle tone occurs, due to a lack of essential mineral salts in the body. Molasses proves most valuable in these cases, as the salts it contains help to re-establish muscle tone.

One distinguished doctor I know was of the opinion that if the sodium salts – which we absorb from our food and from table salt – are not counteracted by potassium salts, there will be a great risk of growths or arthritis developing. If potassium salt is taken into the body daily, it will help in the elimination of sodium salts, and thus minimize the danger. A good, natural way of getting potassium salt into the body is through the taking of crude, black molasses.

Some elderly people are found to have sodium deficiency when they have blood tests. Considering the easy availability of sodium in the diet, this deficiency may owe more to a lack of potassium than a lack of sodium, especially when you consider some of the symptoms of potassium deficiency:

- shortness of breath
- dry, wrinkled, flabby skin
- prolapsed eyelids
- dry mouth
- insomnia,
- irritability
- joint pains
- muscle pains and cramps
- stiffness
- feeling washed out
- itchy, sore eyes that tire easily
- dark circles and bags under the eyes
- depression
- mental fatigue and forgetfulness
- body feeling heavy and tiring easily
- dull and unmanageable hair
- cold hands and feet.

So why does sodium deficiency occur? The body becomes acidic when there are not enough alkaline minerals to balance the acid. Both sodium and potassium are alkaline minerals; potassium is found mostly in the body's cells and sodium mostly in the blood. When the blood becomes too acidic, potassium is drawn out of the cells and into the blood to help, with sodium, to neutralize the excess acid. Sodium is much more plentiful in the modern diet than potassium and so is replenished quickly, while potassium levels get lower and lower. As the potassium is depleted, sodium replaces it in the cells and is therefore found in lower quantities in the blood.

In my view, low blood sodium levels tend to improve if more potassium is made available in the diet to re-establish a proper sodium/potassium balance. This is achieved by taking molasses as well as cider vinegar and honey drinks.

Bathing in Epsom salts

The skin provides an excellent medium for the elimination of acid, and the use of Epsom salts as a 'drawing agent' cannot be too highly recommended. Epsom salts may be obtained from chemists, the pharmacy counter in supermarkets and quite often from garden centres. I believe that roses benefit from the valuable mineral salts it contains. It provides magnesium and sulphur. Magnesium, an alkaline mineral, is quickly and efficiently absorbed into the body through the skin but not necessarily so through the digestive tract. Sulphur combines with toxic acids in the body, converts them to a non-toxic form that is then excreted. Epsom salts provide them both, and there is nothing more relaxing than an Epsom salts bath at the end of a long, painful day. The following method is my particular favourite:

1 Dissolve one pound (or three teacups) of Epsom salts in a bath of water as hot as you can bear it. (It should be noted that patients suffering from angina, high blood pressure, or any heart condition, should not use very hot water.) Do not add soap or bath cubes, salts or oils, as the alkalinity of these products will fight the acidity of the Epsom salts, thereby minimizing its effects.

2 Keep the water hot, by adding more from time to time, and start to exercise your joints. Beginning with the toes move them backwards and forwards; rotate the ankles clockwise and anticlockwise; bend the knees and relax and stretch them; bend the

spine backwards and forwards; bend and move the neck; rotate the arms clockwise and anti-clockwise; then exercise the fingers by clenching and unclenching the hand and then stretching the fingers as wide apart as possible. When exercising the fingers, a gentle, forceful movement is beneficial, as this helps to force out those acid deposits that have accumulated on the bones and between the joints.

3 The heat of the water will open the pores of the skin, enabling the Epsom salts to 'draw out' acid poisons. After ten to fifteen minutes, get out of the bath, dry yourself quickly with a warm towel, and get straight into a warm bed. The object of this is to keep the pores of the skin open all night, to encourage the elimination of acid through sweating. Patients may find that sleeping between blankets will help to absorb the sweat.

This bath is a wonderful relaxer and pain-reliever, and a good night's sleep will usually be achieved. On rising, take a quick shower to wash away the accumulated acids and you will emerge refreshed and ready to face another day. It should be noted that this bath can be slightly weakening, and the patient may feel lethargic the following day. If this occurs, an hour's rest at midday will prove beneficial. For working arthritics, two baths, taken at weekends, may be advisable, and I certainly recommend that no more than three Epsom salts baths be taken per week.

On no account should the body be exposed to cold or draughts after this bath. This could lead to tension in the nerves and muscles, thereby causing pain and making matters far worse than before. Similarly, no work should be undertaken after the bath. Keeping warm is most important, as it will prolong the period of 'elimination'. A methodical 'pinching' of the skin, from the feet upwards, will help to increase circulation and improve muscle tone. However, under no circumstances should this bath lead to exhaustion.

Of course, many arthritics are unable to get into the bath, and I suggest that they bathe hands and feet, as follows:

1 Take an ordinary kitchen bowl, and fill it with water as hot as you can bear.

2 Add to this one cupful of Epsom salts, and soak hands for ten to fifteen minutes.

3 Using forceful but gentle exercise, you will find it amazing how quickly movement is regained in previously locked joints.
4 Dry the hands, and wrap in a warm towel for five minutes to allow the pores to close.
5 Repeat this process with the feet.

These hand and feet baths may be taken three times daily or more often if possible. In many cases, some power will be regained in the hands within six weeks of regular treatment, and patients will find that they have the confidence to get in and out of the bath, without fear of falling. I once had a patient whose hands and fingers had become deformed and locked. In the course of four months of treatment, all this had disappeared. This lady was delighted to tell me that she could now open a tin of dog food without any difficulty. She is just one of the many who are daily experiencing similar results.

Very often, arthritics experience inflammation, pain and swelling in various joints. A cold, wet pack will relieve this in a manner little short of miraculous. This should be carried out as follows:

1 Wring out some linen, or similar material, in cold water.
2 Wrap this around the affected part and cover with a woollen scarf or some warm flannelling.

This application will increase circulation to the affected part and draw out the pain and swelling, without the need to resort to any harmful drug. These natural treatments are often scornfully described as 'old wives' tales'. However, their obvious merits should not be ignored in favour of drugs, which will only do you more harm in the long run.

The self-healing power of the body is really wonderful and nature is the only true healer. No matter what methods of treatment are employed, the body must and always will depend on the 'setting free' of the healing powers and forces within it. The essence of much disease is the accumulation of waste acids in the system, due to wrong dietetic habits and stress. Elimination of these wastes is what nature is striving for, and therefore the tremendous value of the foregoing 'detoxification' programme should be obvious. Remember, good health has to be earned and worked for, but you will find the results well worth achieving.

Avoiding stress

First and foremost, the main requirement for ridding the body of arthritis is positive thinking. This attitude of mind towards the success of the treatment is of paramount importance. Every member of the family can encourage the arthritic sufferer to adopt this attitude, and indeed, the diet that I recommend could prove beneficial to the family as a whole.

The avoidance of stress is also important. Stress is a commonly used term that is rather more easily recognized than explained. Because stress is really a personal condition, it can mean a number of different things to different people. In general, a person can be described as suffering from stress, when the pressures of work, family problems, money worries and so on, get beyond his ability to cope and thus ruin his peace of mind. These conditions invariably lead to impatience, irritability, depression, loss of concentration and sleeplessness.

Stress can also affect a person in a physical manner. Anxiety, fear and worry increase the body's production of chemicals called stress hormones. These can cause feelings of panic or discomfort in a normally healthy person, but to the arthritic, the outcome of the production of these hormones is often more serious. Stress hormones can raise the blood pressure, which in turn may lead to other complications. Stress is nothing new – living has always involved stress – but in recent times problems such as mass unemployment and the nuclear threat, as well as the daily strains of modern living, have greatly increased its effects.

In April 2012, Carnegie Mellon University published a study in the *Proceedings of the National Academy of Sciences*. The study revealed that:

> Stress wreaks havoc on the mind and body . . . with the body losing its ability to regulate the inflammatory response . . . The research shows for the first time that the effects of psychological stress on the body's ability to regulate inflammation can promote the development and progression of disease . . . Runaway inflammation is thought to promote the development and progression of many diseases.

> (*PNAS*, 109 (16), pp. 5995–9)

There is some evidence that those most likely to suffer from stress often display similar personality traits. These people are usually impatient, ambitious, competitive and, as such, under constant pressure. A sudden, severe shock – such as news of a death in the family – has been known to cause a relapse in arthritis.

This is what happened to one of my patients, Lorraine. By the age of 44, Lorraine had many health problems: the pain and inflammation of arthritis since the age of 36, spondylosis/scoliosis, muscle loss, difficulty walking and sitting, headaches, depression, tiredness, memory loss, psoriasis, breathlessness, dizziness . . . she was in trouble. Worried about developing a stomach ulcer, she had stopped taking indometacin and co-proxamol. She had been signed as 'unfit' for work for a year; her employer had suggested that she needed special equipment and that she should apply for funding for it. She was under a great deal of stress, but Lorraine was anxious to return to work. It was April 1992.

Two months into her treatment, her walking no longer felt 'as bad as walking on glass – more like gravel'. Her hay fever and dizziness had improved; the pain was more intermittent; her feet and ankles were much improved; and her headaches had eased off. She no longer needed painkillers – she felt sore but it was bearable. This improvement brought her strength on various levels. She was able to do exercises and go swimming. A gradual improvement meant that one year after starting the treatment, she could 'walk quite rapidly . . . and could even carry shopping . . . I could hardly believe the improvement in my health'. She continued with the treatment and started studying to become a teacher, gaining a diploma in 1996 and finally completing her studies in June 2001.

In March 2001, however, she lost both her parents; she suffered renewed pains in her legs, stiffness in her hands, tiredness and listlessness, and she succumbed to a bout of flu that lasted three weeks – all due to the stress of bereavement. Rather than taking medications, she said 'I am beginning to adopt a more positive approach to everyday life; I do not believe in dwelling on the negatives.' She renewed her efforts with the natural treatment, despite her doctor trying to dissuade her at the very start. When Lorraine spoke to him about the programme, she reported that he wasn't 'happy about what he considers alternative medicine and hit the roof at the mention of cider vinegar and honey'.

Very often, there is no way of knowing if someone is suffering from stress. However, there may be 'tell-tale' signs, for example, heavier smoking and drinking habits, sudden overeating, or loss of appetite. Sleeplessness, unaccountable tiredness, short temper, and an unusual difficulty in making decisions, are also signs of stress. Life is complicated, especially for the arthritic, but we often make matters worse for ourselves. For example, we often put ourselves under tremendous pressure by leaving things to the last possible minute. To avoid this, do everything you can at a reasonable pace, without hurrying. Plan ahead – give yourself plenty of time to shower and dress in the morning, and above all, do try to have a pleasurable, unhurried breakfast. This will ensure a good start to the day and set the pace for the following working hours. It is well worth getting up an hour earlier, in order to achieve this. To help avoid stress:

1 Take plenty of regular exercise, if possible – it is one of the best forms of relaxation.
2 Eat slowly, taking your mind off your work while doing so.
3 Find ways to 'escape' in your spare time, through books, pastimes, hobbies and sport.
4 Make sure you take a regular holiday. Do not make the excuse that you have not got time – make time!
5 Make sure you have enough rest – relaxation is vital. Some light reading at bedtime can help you to 'let go' mentally and physically before you go to sleep.
6 Try to avoid getting over-impatient; few things are that urgent. If you really must get angry about something, try to get it out of your system by expressing your anger as quickly and honestly as possible.
7 Do not bottle up your anger, but try to find ways of getting rid of it.
8 Make sure that the goals you are trying so hard to achieve are what you really want. Ask yourself whether you need to be so competitive.
9 When you are anxious, make a special effort not to smoke or drink any more than usual. This will only be self-defeating in the long run, and the same applies to overeating.

10 Make a positive effort to change the things in your life that are a constant source of worry.

Having started the day supported by the power of positive thinking, you should now turn your thoughts to diet, and the eating of the correct foods necessary to the health of your body.

Rules for healthy eating

To the arthritic, an acid-free diet is of the utmost importance. However, the following dietary 'rules' are of value not only to the arthritic, but also prove beneficial to the overweight and those with heart conditions.

1 *Eat less salt*
Most of us eat much more salt than we need, and for some people, too much salt actually leads to increased blood pressure. Cut down on your salt intake by:

- using less salt in cooking;
- never adding salt to prepared food;
- choosing fresh, rather than processed foods;
- avoiding salty foods, such as crisps, salted peanuts, etc.

2 *Cut out animal fats*
Butter, cheese, milk and cream are very high in lactic acid, and should be avoided altogether. These animal fats provide arachidonic acid, which increases inflammation. Cut down on your intake of fat by:

- using a vegetable spread such as olive oil, sunflower or soya;
- using organic dried or skimmed milk, or almond, nut, oat, rice or soya milk, preferably unsweetened;
- eating cottage cheese – not to be confused with cream cheese, which is very high in lactic acid.

There are different types of helpful fats (or 'essential fatty acids'), which I shall explain later in this chapter.

3 *Cut out all citrus fruits*
Oranges, lemons, grapefruit, and their juices, are full of citric acid. When combined with carbohydrates in the system, the

result is a formation of uric acid. Pineapples, tomatoes, straw-
berries, plums, gooseberries and rhubarb are also high in acids,
as are blackcurrants, redcurrants, blackberries and damsons. This
also applies to fruit jams and marmalades, and to pickles made
with malt or spiced vinegar. As a practical rule of thumb, if you
think of a fruit and your mouth waters, it contains acid and
should be avoided.

Unfortunately, citrus fruits provide a major source of vitamin
C. This vitamin is of vital importance to the body and a lack
of it can create iron deficiency, even leading to anaemia. It is
essential, therefore, to take a good, naturally produced vitamin
C supplement each day, and I will enlarge on this at a later stage.

4   *Cut out 'old meats'*
Pork, beef, ham, bacon, sausages, pâtés, corned beef and similar
prepared meats all contain old, fibrous tissue, full of acid. These
days, when animals have a temperature, stomach upset or minor
ailment, they are pumped with antibiotics and other drugs, just
as we are. When their meat is taken into our system, the residual
'poison' of those drugs is also taken in, thereby setting up more
problems for the already 'toxic' arthritic. Animals also eliminate
acid waste from their bodies in much the same way as we do –
through urination and bodily excretions. When they are killed
for meat, this process of elimination stops suddenly. The acids
seep back into the tissues, and when that meat is ingested, the
animal's acids are ingested with it. The suffering arthritic has
then got double trouble – not only his own toxic acids to get rid
of, but also the acids of those animals as well. It therefore makes
sense to avoid these meats whenever possible.

5   *Cut out alcohol*
All alcoholic drinks are high in acid, and should be avoided.
This applies to all spirits such as whisky, vodka, gin, brandy, port
and sherry, all white, red, rosé and dessert wines, beer, larger
and cider. All carbonated drinks should also be avoided as they
contain carbonic acid, for example lemonade, colas, pop, tonic
water, bitter lemon, ginger ale, soda water, ginger beer, shandy,
and all 'Diet' drinks.

6   *Cut out all fried foods, white sugar and white bread*

7 *Avoid cream cakes and biscuits*

8 *Avoid all fruits bottled in syrup*

Foods for a healthy diet

There are a host of 'healthy' foods available to the arthritic, and it only takes a little thought and planning to ensure a well-balanced and varied diet. The following are some guidelines and suggestions for healthy eating:

1 Always buy 100 per cent wholemeal bread – you will find it more satisfying than white bread, and it is far better for you.

2 Choose an olive oil, sunflower oil or soya spread, or preferably avoid butter and margarine altogether and drizzle extra virgin olive oil or a lighter tasting oil such as flaxseed oil on your bread. We read a lot these days about 'essential fatty acids'. Omega-3 fats, omega-6 fats and omega-9 fats are all essential fatty acids – 'essential' because they are necessary in order to sustain a healthy body. Olive oil is a source of omega-9 fat that has been specifically found to decrease inflammation, so it is very helpful to the arthritis sufferer. Corn oil, nut oil, flaxseed oil and safflower oil are rich in omega-6 fats, which we need to take more of, so these too can be used in the diet. However, as chemicals are often used in their production, it would be prudent to choose only those labelled 'organic'. One of the constituents of an omega-6 fat is a substance called GLA. This is found in evening primrose oil, blackcurrant seed oil and borage oil, which all help to reduce inflammation.

3 Eat no more than three or four eggs per week.

4 Eat fresh, white fish – grilled, poached, baked or steamed, but never fried! Tinned fish, because of its invariably high salt content, is best avoided unless rinsed first. Oily fish should be eaten as it is an important source of omega-3 fat. Constituents of omega-3 fats are eicosapentaenoic acid (EPA) and docosahexaenoic (DHA) – once again relatively new terminology. It is far better to take in these substances in the form of good food than in supplement form. Natural food contains many healthgiving ingredients, some

of which may well have not yet been identified, but those ingredients are synergistically balanced in the right proportions.

5 Eat plenty of cottage cheese, varying it with the addition of chives, spring onions or chopped Spanish onions. Onions are a wonderful blood cleanser and a natural antibiotic. One tablespoon of raisins added to cottage cheese is another variation; also, fresh fruit, excluding of course the ones that contain acid.

At lunch-time after a particularly busy morning in the Clinic, I find that an easy, satisfying, tasty and nourishing meal can be made by adding sliced banana, apple, peach and a few raisins to a tub of natural cottage cheese.

6 Lamb may be eaten in moderation, and of course, the mint sauce can be made with cider vinegar – it tastes delicious! To sweeten the sauce, add one teaspoon of brown sugar or honey.

7 Eat chicken, duck, turkey, or indeed any fowl – although duck, being fatty, is less desirable.

8 Eat rabbit, lamb's liver, and heart. Kidneys, being an eliminative organ, should be avoided.

9 Eat plenty of fresh vegetables, raw or cooked. Salads are most beneficial, but do not add tomatoes, as they have a high acid content. Vegetables, especially leafy greens, are another source of those helpful essential fatty acids. Essential fatty acids help to improve health by increasing energy and stamina, assisting in weight reduction, clearing excess water from the tissues, lowering raised blood pressure, decreasing cravings, reducing depression and improving brain function. One other very important function related specifically to inflammation is that they make blood less sticky, which reduces the possibility of a blood clot forming in an artery or brain, thereby protecting from heart attacks and strokes. Try to have some raw vegetables every day in the form of a salad. As well as two or three vegetables with your main meal of the day, have freshly made vegetable soup too, as often as you can. Make your own and avoid the dried or tinned varieties, since they contain sugar, salt and other preservatives, colourings and flavourings.

10 Choose fruits from among the many types that do not contain citric acid – for example, peaches, pears, bananas, apples, apricots and melons.

11 Drinks, I am afraid, are limited. Apple juice, or any vegetable extract – for example, carrot juice – can be taken, but alcohol should be avoided, if possible. This is a bone of contention with many of my patients. They ask, 'What can I have when I want a drink with my friends?' Beer or Guinness may be the least harmful, or otherwise a small glass of your favoured drink – but only one! If one must have alcohol, it is advisable to take an extra dose of cider vinegar, with or without honey, in order to cope with the extra acid intake. Still apple juice, still mineral water, a cup of tea or coffee, depending on the circumstances, would be good choices. You could offer to be the driver for a night out if you need an excuse to break previous habits. Not only would you be popular in saving your friends' taxi fares, but you health would benefit.

12 Eat plenty of wholemeal cereals, and make your own pastries and cakes with wholemeal flour and oils such as grapeseed or sunflower oil which have little distinctive taste of their own.

13 When buying food read the labels. Be very aware of what the product contains, and if there is anything in it that you should not have or you do not recognize – put it back.

14 Cut down your intake of tea – it is full of tannic acid. If you must drink tea, make it weak. Also, use organic decaffeinated coffee instead of ordinary coffee, which has a very high caffeine content. Hot drinks can be made with herbal teas – there is a wide variety to choose from.

You will find that the feeling of well-being, and the lessening of pain achieved by following these 'dietary rules', will have been well worth any sacrifice and effort involved.

Nutrition

I have found from my clinic that the vast majority of arthritics are extremely undernourished. Most are anaemic and suffer from stress and its related effects. I find that a good short cut to making them feel better is the administration of a variety of vitamins and minerals, as follows:

1 I supply a good, well-balanced range of vitamins and minerals which are specially made for the arthritic, called 'the Margaret Hills Formula'. This introduces a complete range of vitamins and minerals to nutritionally starved bodies. Coupled with 'the Margaret Hills Protein' powder, this is an excellent basis for a return to good health.

2 If patients are anaemic, I give additional iron with vitamin C. If severely anaemic, even more nutrients are introduced.

3 If patients suffer from cramps and tingling sensations, I give extra calcium in tablet form along with co-factors to help absorb it.

4 I always recommend a vitamin C supplement, as the greatest source of this vitamin – citrus fruits – is not allowed.

5 Vitamin B complex is a must, as it feeds and soothes tired nerves, thus promoting a good night's sleep. Many people who come to the clinic already take one or other of the B vitamins, as they have been told that it is good for them. However, they do not realize that the taking of only *one* B vitamin will create a deficiency of the other B vitamins in the body and can, therefore, cause more harm than good.

6 I find concentrated alfalfa extremely useful, and often give it to people who cannot take black molasses. Alfalfa seems to have similar properties and in my experience, very good results have been achieved through its use. Sprouted alfalfa seeds are very good too and can be sprinkled on salads, for example.

As I have stressed, over and over again, arthritis is a disease of dietetic origin, and as such, should be treated accordingly. The following chapter is designed to give the reader a further awareness of the importance of a good, wholesome diet.

4

Vitamins and minerals – their uses in the body

The more you study your nutrition, the more you learn about food, and the more you understand how your body works. Eating a lot does not necessarily mean getting the correct nourishment. More important than quantity is a variety of foods, that contain the correct amounts of proteins, minerals and vitamins needed to supply our bodies with enough energy for growth, repair and maintenance. The consequences may be serious if these vital nutrients are lacking.

Bulk and roughage are very important factors in the foods we eat, because without them the body cannot function properly and a state of acidosis may be set up in our bodies, leading to various chronic ailments.

The adoption of a plan of wholefood nutrition is essential to the good health and efficiency of the human body. When a wound is stitched or a broken bone is manipulated together, we all know that it is the body's own natural healing powers that heal the wound and mend the broken bone. We can also observe these natural healing powers at work in the case of colds or influenza, and in cases of fevers and inflammation. Usually in children and young people this is a very quick process, because at this stage in life the body's resistance is high and depletion of natural powers has not taken place. In older people, the healing is usually slower because the body's natural impetus towards health has been minimized, due to years of inadequate diet, stress and abuse of the body through smoking, excessive alcohol and – inadvertently perhaps – by other pollutants. It is my belief that if all these instances were treated by the whole person elimination treatment which I advocate, not only would there be a swift return to normal health, but the patient would actually feel much better after than he did before the disease or wound occurred. This is because the body would have thrown off those harmful toxic acids and a clean, healthy body would have emerged.

Unfortunately, the long-suffering doctor, when called to the patient's bedside, is expected to perform a miracle and has no alternative but to give the patient a drug or antibiotic selected from the vast array available. The doctor has no time to explain to his patients that self-healing processes will go to work. The patient, however, may think that the GP just can't be bothered if he advises leaving the condition alone; but a programme of intelligent 'leaving alone' may be much better than medical intervention, which could be harmful. For years I have practised in my family a drugless campaign of treatment and this form of the promotion of my children's health has paid dividends. I maintain that a good diet supported by nutritional supplements in the form of protein, vitamins and minerals helps to promote good health and vigour.

Vitamins

'Vitamin' is a term applied to a group of substances which exist in minute quantities in natural food and which are necessary to normal nutrition, especially in connection with growth and development. Vitamin deficiency in the diet of young children and animals causes defective growth. In adults various diseases can arise, and persistent deprivation of one or other vitamin is apt to lead to a lower state of general health. Certain deficiencies in diet, or an inability to metabolize vitamins correctly, have been known to cause all kinds of health problems, scurvy (vitamin C deficiency), beriberi (vitamin B1 deficiency) and rickets (vitamin D, calcium, and other deficiencies).

It is important to realize that vitamins and minerals work hand in hand. They do not appear singly in nature, so taking a supplement of just one vitamin or mineral would be strange to the body and would probably cause a further imbalance of nutrients. For instance, it is known that the mineral zinc releases vitamin A from the liver, where it is stored. So, if someone appears to be lacking vitamin A, it is important to consider zinc deficiency too because a supplement of zinc could be truly what is needed, in order to release the vitamin A already present in the body.

Vitamin A

This vitamin is usually taken in more than ample quantity in a normal diet and is stored in the liver. It is developed originally by plants as a yellow colouring matter – carotene, for example, in carrots. It is found as 'beta-carotene' in colourful fruits and vegetables, and as 'retinol' in animal products such as egg yolk, liver, milk and butter. Children and pregnant women have a higher requirement. Deficiency of vitamin A can be responsible for serious inflammation of the eyes known as 'xerophthalmia'; also for night blindness, various skin eruptions, defective development of the teeth and lack of vitality in the tissues, which could lead to localized inflammation. It is not destroyed by ordinary cooking processes.

Too much vitamin A can be harmful. It has been suggested that more than 1.5 mg of retinol would be too much, and pregnant women should avoid high doses.

Vitamin B1

Constipation, flatulence and dyspepsia can be the result of a mild deficiency of vitamin B1, and such problems lead on to headaches, lack of energy and chronic fatigue. Vitamin B1 is found in the husks of cereals and grains. Its deficiency may be produced by too careful milling of rice or by a diet of white bread to the exclusion of brown bread and other cereal sources of this vitamin. The resulting disease is a form of neuritis, with muscular weakness and heart failure. The best sources of this vitamin are wholemeal flour, bacon, liver, egg yolk, yeast and pulses. Pregnant women require higher amounts. In a healthy body, all the B vitamins can be produced by 'friendly bacteria' in the gut.

Vitamin B2

This is present in milk and is not destroyed during pasteurization. Other rich sources are eggs, liver, yeast and the green leaves of broccoli and spinach. It is also present in beer. Deficiency of this vitamin in the diet is thought to cause inflammation of the cornea, sores on the lips, and dermatitis. Women require higher amounts during pregnancy and lactation. Vitamin B2 is important in combating anaemia – it works with iron and other nutrients to make haemoglobin. Haemoglobin (measured by blood testing) is often lower than it should be in people suffering with arthritis.

Vitamin B3

Vitamin B3, otherwise known as niacin, nicotinic acid or nicotinamide, has been found to lower high cholesterol levels, improve circulation and help with digestion. It is involved in the inflammatory process and helps to relieve pain, improve the mobility of the joints and improve muscle strength. It also helps to ease fatigue. Once again a variety of other substances is necessary for the proper utilization of vitamin B3 in the body so it should not be taken as a single supplement. Vitamin B3 is distributed widely in foodstuffs, both animal and vegetable. Yeast, liver and egg yolk are particularly rich sources.

Vitamin B6

Vitamin B6, the active form being known as pyridoxal-5-phosphate or PLP, plays an important part in the metabolism of a number of amino acids. Deficiency leads to atrophy of the epidermis, the hair follicles and the sebaceous glands; neuritis may also occur. Young infants are more susceptible to deficiency than adults. They may lose weight, develop anaemia, and become very irritable; convulsions may also occur.

Vitamin B6 has come to prominence for its ability to alleviate the pain and depression associated with pre-menstrual syndrome, the nausea of early pregnancy, and post-natal depression. These beneficial effects occur because it can help to control the hormones oestrogen and cortisol in the body. A deficiency of vitamin B6, along with other vital nutrients that work with it, contributes to PMS (premenstrual syndrome), IBS (irritable bowel syndrome) and diseases like multiple sclerosis, schizophrenia and various inflammatory disorders.

Liver, yeast and cereals are rich sources of vitamin B6; fish is a moderately rich source, but milk and vegetables contain little.

Vitamin B12

This vitamin contains cyanide and cobalt. It was first isolated in 1948 and was found to be effective in the treatment of pernicious anaemia. Vitamin B12 is needed for the production of red blood cells. Like the other B vitamins, it is manufactured in the gut, but some people find it difficult to absorb into the blood from the gut – those with thyroid difficulties, for instance – and vegans may require additional amounts. A serious deficiency of vitamin B12 can cause mental illness, neuralgia, neuritis and possibly bursitis. For the proper absorption of vitamin B12, calcium and various other nutrients are required.

Brewers' yeast is one of the richest sources of the B vitamins. Even so, it can take as much as 1 kg of yeast to yield some of the smaller dosages of B vitamins per capsule, currently quoted on the labels of vitamin supplements.

Vitamin C

This is especially found in fresh citrus fruits such as oranges, lemons and grapefruits; also in green vegetables and, to a smaller extent, in milk, meat and other fresh foods. Canned vegetables, such as tomatoes, retain it as their reaction is acid. It is quickly destroyed by high temperature or by excess baking soda and other alkalis, and is gradually lost by oxidation in storage. Its deficiency leads to symptoms of scurvy, including muscular weakness, haemorrhages under the skin, swelling and inflammation of the gums, with loss of teeth, and serious damage to joints by haemorrhage. Vitamin C helps to reduce inflammation. It is a powerful antioxidant that helps fight infections. If a person suffers with allergic reactions, there is an increased requirement for vitamin C. Deficiency can occur in babies fed persistently on artificial foods.

Vitamin D

This vitamin is of special value for the growth of children, and its deficiency produces rickets, with softening and irregular growth of bones, so that swollen joints, distorted limbs, deformities of the chest and similar malformations arise. Deficiency in an adult can lead to osteomalacia and osteoporosis. If you are housebound or have darker skin, or are otherwise not exposed to much sunlight, you are likely to be deficient in vitamin D. Only a few foods contain vitamin D naturally; they include cod liver oil and other fish oils. Egg yolk contains a smaller quantity; fats and milk contain very small quantities. Sunlight acting on the skin is actually the best source of vitamin D for the body. This vitamin aids in the absorption of phosphorus and calcium from the food, and increases absorption of these substances into the blood and bones. Bad effects may follow overdosage, because if too much calcium and phosphorus are maintained in the blood, the bones and teeth may become overcalcified and unduly hardened and calculi may form in the kidneys and other organs. Supplements are helpful for infants and nursing mothers and those not accessing sunlight routinely.

Vitamin E

Vitamin E is an antioxidant found in seeds, wholegrains, wheatgerm, green leafy vegetables, butter and other fresh foods; it is actually a complex of eight compounds called tocopherols and tocotrienols. It is readily stored in the body and is unlikely to be deficient in human beings, except in cases of very severe undernourishment and in premature babies. Miscarriages may occasionally be due to its deficiency.

Vitamin E is beneficial for the heart, circulation, nerves and muscles and for those with varicose veins. As an antioxidant, it helps to reduce the unnecessary absorption of some harmful substances called 'free radicals'. As with other nutrients, vitamin E does not act in isolation – selenium has been found to enhance its activity in the body.

Vitamin K

This is the anti-haemorrhage vitamin, essential for the proper clotting of blood. It has been given successfully in cases of bleeding in infants and in cases of jaundice where there is a special tendency to bleeding. Bleeding in these conditions is thought to be directly due to deficiency in vitamin K. It is widespread in nature, the main sources being fermented foods such as yoghurt, kefir, kombucha, sauerkraut, sourdough bread, and pickles. Alfalfa, spinach, leafy vegetables, tomatoes and liver provide small amounts. The daily requirement has not been identified. Intestinal micro-organisms – 'friendly bacteria' – synthesize a considerable amount of it. However, it is a fat-soluble vitamin so dietary fat is also required for it to be absorbed properly. Research shows that vitamin K has a significant effect on bone density, helps to prevent hardening of the arteries and slows the growth of cancer cells; deficiency may contribute to the onset of Alzheimer's disease, but it should not be taken as a supplement by anyone who has suffered a stroke or heart attack or is otherwise prone to blood clotting.

Iron

This mineral is an essential constituent of the red blood corpuscles, where it is present in the form of haemoglobin and carries vital oxygen around the body. It is also present in muscle and is essential to the life of many tissues in the body. Adolescents, women with heavy periods, vegetarians, pregnant women, infants and those who undergo strenuous exercise are all prone to iron deficiency. Iron salts have an astringent action, especially the chloride, and sometimes this property is made use of when it is used as a styptic to stimulate blood clotting. Iron helps in building a strong immune system and is better utilized in the body when given alongside vitamin C and the B vitamins. Foods rich in iron include dark meats, liver, egg yolk, lentils and wholegrains.

Calcium

This is an alkaline mineral present in chalk and other forms of lime. It is one of the most important minerals for human health. Calcium along with phosphorus builds strong bones, nails and teeth. Calcium is especially needed by the growing child and the pregnant and nursing mother.

The human body contains more calcium than any other mineral but its absorption is very inefficient and, when the body is under stress, absorption of calcium is even less. To improve calcium absorption, it is vital that the gastric acid secretions in the stomach are optimal. Calcium is widely available in the diet, but rather than relying on milk and cheese, calcium is better obtained from green leafy vegetables such as lettuce and broccoli, as well as seeds (where it is accompanied by magnesium). If calcium is taken in supplement form, it, like other minerals, should not be taken alone. It is not found alone in nature, and for proper absorption, a whole variety of nutrients is necessary, including magnesium, phosphorus, vitamin D, vitamin K, essential fatty acids, protein, vitamin A and vitamin C.

Magnesium

This is one of the essential mineral elements in the body, without which it cannot function properly. Magnesium is generally found in foods such as green leafy vegetables, whole grains, nuts and seeds, avocado, soya beans and soya flour. It has a calming influence on muscles and nerves. One of its most important functions in the body is to balance calcium. Inadequate magnesium means that calcium is not used properly, which can result in muscular weakness, heart-muscle spasms (which can result in angina and arrhythmia), spasms in artery muscle (which can lead to high blood pressure), arthritis, osteoporosis, hardening of the arteries, senility, diabetes, and so on. In addition, common symptoms of inadequate magnesium include indigestion, heartburn and fatigue. A good way to increase magnesium status is via the skin. Magnesium sulphate, commonly known as Epsom salts, is a saline purge, but used in the bath is highly effective in increasing magnesium levels. These baths also help in the elimination of acids from the body, especially in cases of arthritis and rheumatism, and in fact any chronic diseases, such as bronchitis or non-allergic asthma.

Choosing the right foods

Some people acquire dietary habits peculiar to their own fads and fancies, generally relying upon a large amount of filling foods, in complete ignorance of the known principles of nutrition. These habits may have a hereditary influence, because if a mother has not been sufficiently educated in the science of nutrition, to supply her family with healthy food, then there is very little hope that her daughter or son will be taught correct feeding habits, and so the story repeats itself.

In years gone by the bone-deforming disease of rickets was widespread in children throughout their formative years. Their diets were sadly lacking in the fruits and vegetables that provide vitamins and essential mineral salts, and in the absence of these foods, fevers raged and child mortality was high. Large quantities of nutritionally deficient foods are eaten today. The supermarket shelves are full of them and resistance to a change of diet is very persistent. Most of the deficiency foods are fattening and they tend to induce overeating. The refined carbohydrates are of this type – white flour, in its many forms of bread, cakes, pastries, biscuits and pastas, and polished white rice. The modern milling process means that the bran and germ of the wheat are rejected; the nutritionally rich parts of the wholegrain are excluded from the flour, and are sold separately as animal food or breakfast cereal. In this process there is a loss of valuable vitamins and minerals, especially those of the B complex, and also a loss of protein. Natural iron and calcium are among the minerals that are lost but now, iron is added to white flour in another form, as well as chalk to replace the absent calcium. It is stated that as many as 20 chemicals may be used in the production of the modern loaf of white bread. Such chemicals include bleaching agents to whiten the flour, preservatives, texturizers, anti-infection agents, emulsifiers and moisturizing agents. They disrupt the natural mineral balance in the body. The white loaf is no longer the 'staff of life'. It is better to buy flour and bread that is 100 per cent freshly baked organic wholemeal, but where digestive problems are present, 'sprouted wheat' bread is better still.

The well-being of the consumer depends entirely on the consumption of food in its pure natural state. In the case of flour, as with all other foods, it is a complex combination of substances that, when tampered with and some of the vitamins removed, is likely to be rendered completely valueless in terms of nutrition.

There is a direct relation between the consumption of wholefoods and the control of rheumatism and arthritis, and the springing up of wholefood shops around the country is not surprising. The problem remains that, although there is a crying need for wholefood nutrition, the public at large are ignorant of their requirements and do not know what to buy for their various illnesses. They buy vitamin E or whatever, because a friend told them it is good. Good for what, they don't know and have no idea of where to find out. A resident nutrition practitioner well versed in the uses of vitamins and minerals would be a tremendous boon, both to the health food store and the customer. People want to be healthy, but they don't know how to go about achieving that happy state.

White sugar is another threat to good nutrition. By the year 1700 the commercial refining of sugar had made it readily available and the consumption was 14 lb per person per year. By 1800 the figure had risen to 16 lb per person per year, and at present it runs at about 150 lb per person per year. This commodity cannot be classed as food because it is completely devoid of all vitamins and minerals. One can become addicted to it; its chemical formula is not unlike that of alcohol. Sugar is a refined carbohydrate and dentists everywhere tell us that it is the principal cause of dental caries. It can be responsible for a vast array of other diseases, including obesity, diabetes, diseases of the intestine such as those very often found in conjunction with arthritis – colitis and diverticulitis; also constipation, haemorrhoids and varicose veins. All of these are blood disorders and directly related to rheumatism and arthritis.

Honey is often preferred to sugar because it is a more natural product than refined sugar. It has fewer calories, too – about 82 per ounce, compared with 112 for sugar. Analysis also shows that honey contains traces of many minerals and trace elements and some samples of honey also contain vitamins. To produce honey, the bee has partly digested complex sugars into simpler glucose and fructose sugars that are less disruptive to human blood sugar levels. Because honey is a natural product many health food shops carry a large selection. Taste is often the deciding factor in purchasing a particular type of honey. For those who like a light-coloured honey with a delicate flavour, acacia is a good choice. Set honey is traditionally used with teatime bread and butter, or breakfast toast. Liquid honey is easier for cooking or for use in drinks, remedies or natural beauty recipes. If you use honey for cooking it is best to choose one with a subtle flavour that will not overpower the other ingredients, and remember that honey is 20 per cent water.

Blended honey is the cheapest, because it is usually the product of more than one country. The most expensive honeys are single source honeys. These are produced by bees that have collected nectar wholly or mainly from one type of flower. The nectars give the honeys very distinctive flavours and colours.

'Pure' honey on a label means that the jar contains 100 per cent honey, even though it is blended, as opposed to a 'honey spread' product that contains sugar, syrups and other additives. Honey is the natural replacement for sugar – and much more beneficial to health.

Constructing a well-balanced diet

Disease is exactly what it says – DIS-EASE, and this means that for one reason or another the body is not *at ease*. If I cut my finger my whole body is in sympathy with that finger. Depending on the severity of the cut, there is a sudden shock, which will probably affect my nerves, giving me sleepless nights, which in turn will render me devoid of all energy and as a result my work will suffer. The reader will deduce from this statement that one simple action can bring about a chain of events, each one more serious than the other. In like manner, if we give a sweet, cake or pastry as a reward to a child for a job well done, or to stop him crying, it can trigger off a chain of events that may take years to come to fruition.

Similar symptoms may be related to a variety of conditions, most or all directly related to degenerative conditions in the body due to years of faulty dieting. Orthodox medical methods of treatment in the cure of arthritis and rheumatism have been unsuccessful because these diseases are systemic, due to years of inadequate diet, and nobody will succeed in the treatment of these diseases without an all-round promotion of health. There is no standard diet suitable for all individuals and identifying what is and what is not needed in any particular diet and supplemental nutrient pattern requires more than guesswork; although there is always an element of trial and error initially. Skilled observation, backed by extensive knowledge, chance observations using clues from questions and from the nutrient content of existing diets, experimentation with dietary improvement and nutritional supplements are all ways of determining a patient's nutritional deficiency. To rely on dietary adjustment alone when dealing with specific and unique needs of sick individuals, and to ignore the proven need for supplementation, is a futile exercise. I believe very strongly in supplementation, and I also believe in explaining in detail to my patients what various vitamin supplements will achieve for them. In alternative medicine as in life, it is by our fruits that we shall be known and judged.

Healing is really a very simple affair calling for love, discernment, wisdom and truth. The more complicated treatments are, the harder they are to understand and stick to. Hippocrates said that foods should be medicines and medicines food, and the true practitioner will discuss with his patient what foods, for whatever reasons, are poisonous to him. The practitioner may see the supplement as a nutrient but not so the patient who, in my experience, often sees it as a prop or substitute for balanced nutrition.

It should be clear from all this that there is nothing to equal a well-balanced diet. Experts say we must reduce intakes of fat, sugar and ordinary salt, and take more bread, potatoes, fresh vegetables and fruit. This is true no doubt, but you might add the considerations of quality and selection. *What kind of bread?* one may ask; we have to be careful with brown bread – it may have additives. *How were the vegetables grown?* Have they been sprayed or chemical fertilizers added? If so they may be completely devoid of the vitamins and minerals that are attributed to them. We should look to the fruit we eat: some people never eat fruit and this applies especially to arthritics, who cannot take citrus fruits. Here again it seems evident that some food supplements are necessary to our modern society. According to a report commissioned by the British Government from a group of doctors and scientists, we need more wholefoods, real bread, fresh vegetables and fruit. What these present-day scientists are saying, in effect, is 'we are what we eat'. It seems to me that a gradual change is taking place in public thinking today, and despite the brainwashing of television and other advertising campaigns, the public are beginning to question the value of the average British diet, becoming more selective in their purchase of food and more aware of the ingredients it contains.

It takes a long time to adapt the body to any new or altered system of diet. If you are new to wholefoods, you should change to any new diet gradually. It is not necessarily wise to change your habits abruptly. The sensible plan is to move slowly and adapt to a natural diet by eating more and more foods that are not much altered from their natural state.

Meat

Meat is one of the foods most altered from its natural state by today's methods of factory farming. If you eat meat, quality – how the animals were reared, fed and slaughtered – must be of prime consideration.

Chicken

One ounce of roast lean chicken gives 6.2 g protein, 1.4 g fat, 54 calories and no carbohydrate. Chicken is high in protein, low in fat and a very good source of iron and nicotinic acid. Vitamins B1 and B2 are also present.

The nutritional value of turkey is similar to that of chicken. Guinea fowl is also low in fat, while duck and goose are distinctly fatty. To lessen the fat content, remove the skin before eating roast meat.

Lamb

The leanest lamb has only about 8 per cent fat. An ounce of lean roast lamb has only about 55 calories. Lean lamb is a very good source of iron.

Veal

Veal is extremely lean, and is a very good buy for arthritics and the health conscious. A 3 oz portion of veal has only 100 calories, but when roasted or fried, it has about 160. Lean veal has the same amount of protein and B vitamins as lean beef, but only half the iron.

There is nothing to equal a well-balanced diet to ensure bodily health and mental vigour, and in searching for a healthy way of eating, many people decide to cut down on the amount of meat they eat and find some other sources of protein.

Fish

Fish has a lot to offer. It may still be an animal food, but the fat it contains is polyunsaturated, unlike that of other animal products. Polyunsaturated fatty acids have been shown to have a beneficial effect on the fats in the bloodstream. Their presence helps to reduce the deposit of saturated fats causing narrowing and hardening of the arteries and contributing to heart disease. Fish, in particular oily fish, like mackerel and herring, offer special types of marine oils that make the blood less likely to form clots which cause thrombosis in the narrowed arteries. Both oily fishes and white fish contain valuable vitamins A and D. White fish need extra oil or liquid added during cooking, but oily fishes do not because their oil content enables them to 'cook themselves'. Wrapped in spinach to keep the steam in and prevent them from drying, they make an excellent and very easy meal. Research has shown that the dramatic drop in the amount of fish eaten in Britain can be correlated to the rise in heart disease. Populations like the Inuit who eat large amounts of seal meat are free from heart disease.

Although fish provides protein, it does not provide fibre, and as a lack of this prevents the bowel functioning properly, some form of fibre should be added to the meal – for example, vegetables or fruit, or both. It is wise to vary the type and size of fish you eat, rather than just sticking to tuna or salmon, for example.

Porridge

Porridge made from oats helps to regulate both blood sugar levels and fats. So porridge is now being recommended for the treatment of diabetes, and in some cases for prevention of diabetes, high blood pressure and heart disease. Oats contain a gummy substance – beta glucans – which is very evident when you are boiling them up yourself. This can apparently reduce blood cholesterol levels by a third, as well as reducing blood sugar and fats. Oat bran is particularly rich in this fibre-based material and porridge oats, being the whole rolled oats, contain all of its natural fibre. Dr James King of the University of Kentucky says of the work being done on oats and porridge:

> This is the first time that anyone has demonstrated that a particular food can lower blood cholesterol. It is not uncommon for someone to come into our hospital with a blood cholesterol count of 300, and go out with a level of 195, which is relatively safe.

When the gummy fibre from oats reaches the colon, it is fermented by bacteria which produce fatty acids. These acids are absorbed into the bloodstream and have the effect of shutting down the body's production of sugar (glucose), which is made from starch and fats. This action lowers and stabilizes the level of blood sugar, a result which is, of course, especially beneficial to diabetics. In any case, oats have traditionally been known as a food for stamina and strength. This new work underlines the value of this important cereal in any really healthy diet. From now on we should look at porridge with the reverence that our forefathers did, and perhaps we would be much healthier for doing so.

Fibre

Bran is the richest source of all dietary fibres. A fibre-rich diet, including bran, is highly desirable, and acts as a preventive measure against diverticulitis. This is a disease of the colon and constipation is now recognized as its underlying cause; bran is very often used in the treatment of diverticulitis. Any dietary substance which retards the absorption of carbohydrates may be beneficial to the body, and in this respect dietary fibre is seen to be a very valuable commodity. A large proportion of people develop difficulty in utilizing carbohydrates in their diets during middle age. This difficulty is caused by a fault in the insulin production of the body. Insulin is known to control excess blood sugar and if this rises too high, sugar appears in the urine and the person is diagnosed as diabetic. A group very closely related to diabetics is the group classified as having 'impaired glucose tolerance'. Lack of dietary fibre may also be the cause of varicose veins, due to abdominal pressure caused by straining when constipated, and also haemorrhoids, for the same reason. Dietary fibre plays a very beneficial role in the stabilizing or correction of these ailments.

A fibre-rich diet for children encourages mastication of food and helps to keep the teeth clean. The old saying 'an apple a day keeps the doctor away' is proved today to be a very wise saying; it does keep the doctor away, and the dentist too. An apple is a wonderful source of fibre. An adequate intake of all nutrients is essential for health and activity, and there are additional requirements for growth, pregnancy, lactation and in times of stress, such as infection. The exact amounts needed are different for each individual, and depend not only on such readily quantifiable factors as height, weight and sex, but also on physical activity throughout the day, the rate of internal activities such as heart beat, and the climate.

I hope that the reader will now be convinced that a good, healthy diet is the essence of physical well-being, and realize that without it, the body will go into a state of dis-ease. 'Prevention is better than cure,' the saying goes – how true. Once the body reaches that sad state of disease, a very determined effort is needed to help it to regain that happy state of profound health that is its birthright. To sum up, I remind you that a daily diet for healthy living should contain the following:

Protein The material of life, found in meats, poultry, fish and dairy products. Soya, as found in tofu, is also a valuable source of protein. In my treatment for arthritis, in which I advocate no red meats or dairy products, a daily intake of soya protein isolate is recommended. However, as long-term effects on the health of the human body have yet to be established, it would be sensible to avoid a routine intake of a protein supplement made from genetically modified (GM) crops. Soya is one of those crops subjected to genetic modification.

Fats To support skin, glandular and brain function, improve healing and keep us warm. Found in fish, avocado, nuts, seeds, beans, olives, and in unfiltered, cold-pressed olive, safflower, sunflower, hemp seed or flaxseed oils, which can be put on salads. Coconut oil or a little olive oil can be used for frying. In the form of polyunsaturated oils – corn oil, peanut oil, etc. Plants are the best wholefood source of polyunsaturated fats.

Carbohydrates To supply us with heat and energy; taken in the form of bread, potatoes, rice and pastas.

Vitamins, minerals and trace elements To enhance immunity, prevent disease and support optimal health. From fresh vegetables and fruit, nuts and seeds.

Roughage or fibre To provide energy and promote good elimination of wastes. From sea vegetables, apples, green vegetables, peas, beans, whole grains and molasses.

The whole person elimination treatment, which I referred to early on, I have practised in my family for years. When any of the family developed influenza or bronchitis, I treated them as follows, with excellent results:

Two days on orange juice only. Two days on fresh fruit only.
On the fifth day, fresh fruit plus half a glass of milk for breakfast, lunch and dinner.
    On the sixth day a little wholemeal bread was introduced and green salad; and from then on a gradual resumption of normal diet.

In the case of lung congestion an Epsom salts bath is invaluable. This bath draws the congestion away from the lungs and, as I said before, it is an excellent medium for eliminating wastes by drawing them out through the skin. The patient gets instant relief.

Vegetarian and vegan diets

Many of my patients are either vegetarian or true vegans. In my opinion, vegetarian and vegan diets are extremely good for lowering high cholesterol in the blood and reducing weight and this in turn will help with the prevention of strokes, heart attacks and the formation of kidney stones. Diabetics, too, benefit from no-meat diets because the high fibre content of a vegetable-rich vegetarian diet slows down the absorption of sugar into the blood, thereby stabilizing the blood sugar level.

Meat is acid-forming. It does contain protein but because most animals are fed all sorts of fattening substances, antibiotics, etc., the residual acids of those products are contained in the meat. Fresh, raw fruit and vegetables, nuts, seeds, pulses and milk, however, contain all the vitamins, minerals and trace elements essential for good nutrition, plus the enzymes with which to digest them. These foods are where you find the largest quantity of all these factors in their most easily accessible and digestible form.

Vegetable protein has a high biological value because of its alkalinity and freedom from saturated fat and cholesterol. Protein is made up of amino acids and it is the proportion and quality of these which determine whether a protein food is valuable or not. Meat and other animal-derived food is first-class protein but the amino acids from both vegetables and fruit produce a higher biological value and are therefore not needed in such quantities.

The fat content of meat varies greatly but it is the excessive amount of omega-6 fat that is the important factor to consider. Excessive omega-6 in the body promotes inflammation. The ideal ratio of omega-3 to omega-6 fats in the diet should be 1:1. In wild animals and grass-fed beef, it is 1:2, but in most meat on sale it is between 1:5 and 1:13. Such meat also delivers more calories and more saturated fat than grass-fed beef. Vegetables, fruit, nuts and seeds, on the other hand, contain mostly unsaturated fat, and even more importantly, supply the essential fatty acids which the body cannot manufacture itself.

Last, but not least, we come to the problem of the metabolic wastes in meat. Meat starts to putrefy the moment it is killed and that process goes on until it is inedible. You eat it in whatever state of decomposition it happens to be. That is the first point. Second, when the animal was killed, it was pouring adrenalin into its bloodstream out of fear of what was about to take place. Too much adrenalin is dangerous and the body had to eliminate it, but in this case there was no time. Third, you consume with meat the various antibiotics and drugs which have been given to the animal and not eliminated. Finally, meat and most animal foods are acid forming and it is those acids which, if allowed to accumulate, cause trouble. Vegetables, on the other hand, are mostly alkaline in their reaction. Having noted all these points, it would seem a logical choice to become a vegetarian.

I do not wish to present a dogmatic approach to vegetarianism – a lot of people would not find it easy to follow. This is the reason that my diet for arthritics includes fish, chicken and lamb. In my opinion, these are the least toxic meats and I think that a compromise is well worth adopting. When I ask vegetarians, who visit the Clinic on appointment, where they get their protein from, a lot are very vague as to what they should be having. They do not eat meat and it stops there. This is a worrying situation and, I believe, contributes to their arthritic condition. Protein should constitute an essential part of the diet as a source of energy, and for the replacement of protein lost in the wear and tear of daily life.

Other sources of protein are milk, eggs, pulses and soya. The milk that is usually available creates more problems than it solves. It is pasteurized and homogenized, which destroys the vitamins and the lactase enzyme necessary to digest it properly. It is from grain-fed cattle and contains residues of fertilizers, herbicides and antibiotics. Pasteurized milk impedes calcium absorption and is associated with an increased risk of bone fractures. Clean, fresh, raw organic milk from free-range, grass-fed cows that is not pasteurized or homogenized promotes health in children, but it has to be sought out at the farm gate. Eggs, each of which contains the material necessary to form a chicken, contain the building material for the formation of bone and muscle in an easily digestible form. Cage-raised chickens though are treated with antibiotics, and in consuming the chicken or the egg, one also consumes traces of antibiotics. Fresh eggs from free-range chickens have a more beneficial nutrient profile. One egg corresponds in nutritive value to approximately 1 oz of meat. Pulses, of which the chief are peas, beans and lentils, have been called 'poor man's beef' because they are cheap and low in fat (hence the habit of eating them combined with fat foods). All my vegetarian patients have a good protein powder in conjunction with their supplements. This strengthens their muscles and feeds their complete system. All vegetarians should take double the prescribed amount of protein so that they are not lacking in this valuable body builder.

5

Recipes for arthritis sufferers

The power of positive thinking is invaluable in getting rid of any disease and arthritis is no exception. Always remember to direct your thoughts away from the fact that you have got arthritis, and instead direct them towards achieving good health. Every morning when you wake up think, 'This is another day, when I have another opportunity to make myself feel better.' Picture yourself as radiantly healthy and then go all out to achieve it, especially through your diet.

Eating the acid-free way is healthy for the whole family and especially for those suffering from heart trouble, high blood pressure or angina, because an acid-free diet is very similar to a low-fat diet, except that citrus fruits and fruit juices are forbidden. However, there is a whole host of foods that you can have without feeling deprived. Healthy eating certainly need not be boring.

Remember to keep away from saturated fats. These are easy to recognize as they remain hard at room temperature – lard, suet, butter, dripping, white cooking fat, hard margarine and, of course, fat from meat.

The fat contained in cheese, cream and milk is exactly the same as the fat contained in butter – it is saturated. Cream cheeses and hard cheeses such as Stilton and Cheddar are very rich in fat, as are double cream and whipping cream. Shop-bought biscuits, pastries, cakes, puddings, sauces and soups invariably contain a very high content of fat. Some vegetable margarines are also highly saturated, so it is wise to read all labels and be aware of what any product contains before you buy it.

The following are ways of cutting down on saturated fat:

1 Cut out all dairy products – butter, cheese, milk and cream.
2 Use skimmed raw milk, soya milk, almond milk or rice milk in tea, coffee or in any recipe demanding milk.

3 Always try to choose cottage cheese. This is very good because, although the fat has been taken away, it contains proteins, vitamins and minerals. However, a little low-fat cheese now and again, maybe once a week, could vary the monotony.

4 Before you cook meat, cut away all obvious fat.

5 Use sunflower margarine, or an olive oil spread, or drizzle a lightly-flavoured oil such as flaxseed or rapeseed as a substitute for butter. Try cottage cheese, hummus, nut butters and seed butters rather than dairy butter.

6 Make your own pastries, cakes and biscuits, using the above where the recipe advises hard margarine or butter.

7 Use coconut or rapeseed oil for basting roasts and grills, for browning meat and vegetables, and for mixing sauces. Salad dressings can be made with mainly extra virgin cold-pressed unfiltered olive, flaxseed or grapeseed oil with a little walnut oil or sesame oil for flavour.

8 Include some oily fish in your menus, but always remember to drain excess oil from canned fish such as tuna, sardines and salmon, herrings and mackerel, because it is added oil and not the polyunsaturated oil from the fish. It is better when buying canned fish to choose fish in brine so that the natural oils do not leach into the added oil. Rinse the fish before use.

9 Go for plain or dry-roasted nuts if you can find them, but don't indulge in cashews, coconuts or salted crisps and peanuts.

Eggs are not a good alternative to meat and fish and three eggs a week are adequate for people with any form of blood disorder. Remember to count all the hidden eggs in the dishes you prepare – i.e. in cakes, puddings and sauces.

Casseroling is a good cooking method: the flavours of the ingredients have time to mellow and you can skim off every trace of fat when the casserole is cold. Use puréed root vegetables – carrots, parsnips, potatoes – as thickeners; they do much less damage than cream or egg yolks.

When eating out, keep your menu simple – fresh fruit is a good starter, or consommé. It is best to avoid creamy soups, pâtés, shellfish, or anything fried. Chicken, fish, or lamb are good for a main course. Always avoid fried foods or pastries – they will probably be prepared with saturated fat. Finish your meal with sorbet or fruit. A little meringue without cream would be acceptable, or different kinds of fresh fruit, though not citrus fruits.

A fresh green salad every day is a must for the arthritic, plenty of lettuce, spring onions or Spanish onions, radishes, green and red peppers, chicory, celery, grated carrot, grated cabbage, etc. Add some natural cottage cheese and a tasty home-made dressing and you have a delightful, health-giving meal.

There is no need to make any radical changes in your eating habits – just eat wholesome foods that contain as much goodness as possible and the least amount of harmful acids, such as tannic acid from tea and coffee. Switch to herbal teas and organic decaffeinated coffee; if you must have tea or coffee, have it weak. It is most important also to avoid lactic acid, the main sources of which are butter, cheese, milk and cream; also, of course, the citric acid contained in citrus fruits and juices and, in fact, any acid fruit. When struggling with poor health or a chronic condition, it pays to nourish ourselves as best we can by eating the best food we can obtain. Most people today are beginning to take a second look at the food they eat and are becoming very aware of what is printed on the label.

Organically grown food – fresh fruit, vegetables, meat, poultry, eggs and milk – is nutritionally superior to non-organic food because it is free from contaminants that burden the body. Nationwide box delivery schemes and food from farmer's markets can be excellent value. However, fresh non-organic food is better than wilted organic food or indeed none at all.

A good breakfast

As I carry out my daily work in the Clinic I meet a lot of patients with digestive problems – hiatus hernia, stomach ulcers, diverticulitis. When I ask them to give me a run down on their daily diet, invariably I am told: 'I never have breakfast; perhaps I will have a cream cracker and a little cheese for lunch, but I always have a good large evening meal when the family come home.' The habit of eating one big meal a day, and especially in the evening, is all wrong. It is an excellent way of raising the blood pressure and putting up blood fats. A protein-rich breakfast will stop that sinking feeling by raising the blood sugar and keeping one alert, thereby giving a good energy output and a feeling of being able to cope with the day's stresses and strains. Wholegrain unprocessed cereal with a little dried fruit, skimmed or powdered milk and the addition of bran is quite delicious and very satisfying. Later in this chapter I will give a selection of nourishing breakfasts. Eating is a very necessary part of living and it is most important that we enjoy what we eat. Getting up an hour earlier in the morning pays dividends. It takes the tension out of the beginning of the day and provides us with enough time to sit down and have a leisurely breakfast, masticating the food properly without having to keep an eye on the time. Of course, wholefood eating cuts out 'empty' calories and provides the body with what it needs to burn up excess fat. Changes in diet need self-discipline, but the rewards are many.

A lot of people drink cup after cup of tea in the morning, but as this stimulates the secretion of gastric juices it should be avoided by people suffering from stomach ulcers. The digestion of starch is delayed in the stomach by the taking of too much tea; also, of course, it is full of tannic acid and for arthritics in particular, this is most undesirable.

Coffee contains a drug called caffeine which in my opinion is an unnatural stimulus for the heart. It dilates the blood vessels in the skin so people suffering from inflamed skin conditions should avoid it altogether. Glaucoma sufferers should not take it because it affects the blood vessels in the eyes. Addiction to coffee is not unusual; I had a female patient in the clinic a short time ago who has nine strong cups of coffee a day – she looked horrified when I asked her to cut it down. She told me that she had run out of her favourite brand about a week previously and experienced tremors, high temperature, migraine, irritability and nervousness. She couldn't go to bed without borrowing some coffee from a friend – then she recovered and her symptoms vanished. Ground coffee contains about 150 mg of caffeine; instant coffee contains about 90 mg. I always advise my patients to switch to organic decaffeinated coffee which only contains about 3 mg, and I also advise herbal teas, some of which are delicious and a very beneficial alternative.

In the following pages you will find a variety of breakfast dishes that can safely be adopted by the arthritic or the heart sufferer. I put porridge oats first as a breakfast – a natural food and still one of the cheapest, yet one of the most wholesome and well-balanced foods available for children and adults alike. Porridge is easily prepared, involving very little effort and furnishing the arthritic with a good, warming start to the day.

Note

In the following recipes, it is necessary to avoid lactic acid, which is present in the creamy portion of cow's milk, as well as goat's and sheep's milk. So where milk is mentioned, use skimmed milk, soya, rice, oat or almond milk, or reconstituted skimmed powdered milk. Lactic acid is also present in butter, which is made from the fat content of milk. Avoid dairy butter as much as possible. Although 'organic' dairy butter has a good balance of essential fatty acids, the lactic acid inhibits its routine use in the acid-free diet. Instead of using dairy butter as a spread, use drizzled extra virgin olive oil, whole-nut butter, seed butter, or organic olive oil, organic sunflower or organic soya spreads. Avoid any margarine or spread containing 'partially hydrogenated vegetable oil', 'hydrogenated fats', 'vegetable shortening' or 'trans-fatty acids'. However, when baking a cake, for example, organic butter may be used because the portion size and therefore the total intake of lactic acid would probably be of little consequence.

Basic breakfast

Porridge

To make porridge, stir one cupful of porridge oats into a saucepan containing three cups of milk or water. Add 1 teaspoon sea salt and bring to the boil, stirring continuously; then simmer for four minutes, stirring occasionally. The porridge is now ready to serve. One or two teaspoons of molasses sugar may be added if desired.

Egg

A poached, boiled or oven-baked whole egg on toast with spread is a nourishing start to the day.

Cereal

A glass of apple juice, or some stewed apple, with a little muesli, is a good idea. Follow this with wholemeal bread rolls, toast or bran muffins spread with honey or nut butter.

Fresh fruit

A pleasant alternative for breakfast is a carton of natural 'live' or 'bio' yoghurt and fresh fruit in season.

Breakfast kipper

Fill a large jug with boiling water. Place the kipper in head first, with the tail just above the surface of the water. Leave for 6 minutes. Serve with wholemeal bread and a healthy spread.

Breakfast recipes

Breakfast Sunshine

4 tablespoons rolled oats	*2 oz sultanas*
1 banana, sliced	*1 oz almonds, chopped*
1 tablespoon honey	*Skimmed milk*
1 teaspoon sunflower oil	

Method Mix all ingredients together and serve with skimmed milk. Serves two.

Bran Muffins

4 oz wholemeal flour	*½ oz soft brown sugar*
2 teaspoons baking powder	*1 egg, size 4*
½ teaspoon sea salt	*½ pint approx. milk*
3 oz bran	*4 tablespoons sunflower oil*
1 tablespoon wheatgerm	

Method Brush 12 deep bun tins with oil. Place dry ingredients in a bowl. Beat egg in a basin with milk and oil. Add to dry ingredients and mix together. Fill each bun tin with the mixture and bake in hot oven, 200°C (400°F), gas mark 6, for 25–30 minutes. Serve warm with spread or honey if desired.

Honey Muesli

2 tablespoons rolled oats
1 apple, grated
1 tablespoon honey

½ cup natural yoghurt or
    milk
Chopped nuts

Method Mix all ingredients together, stirring well, and serve immediately. Makes two servings. Instead of oats other cereals may be used; cracked wheat, barley kernels or some wheatgerm may be added, sunflower seeds, raisins or slices of banana.

Oatmeal Breakfast Cakes

2 oz rolled oats
1 oz plain flour
¼ teaspoon bicarbonate of soda
½ pint milk

1 egg
1 teaspoon clear honey
Coconut or olive oil for frying

Method Mix together the dry ingredients. Beat egg with honey. Stir egg mixture into dry ingredients, then slowly add milk, stirring well. Heat a little oil in a frying pan and drop in tablespoons of the pancake batter, spaced well apart. Cook over a moderate heat. When the top is just set and underside golden, turn and cook the second side. Serve hot with spread or honey. These pancakes make a pleasant change from the usual breakfast toast. Makes 18–20 pancakes. The mixture can be refrigerated for two days. Whisk it well before use.

Fruit Salad

1 apple, chopped
1 sliced banana
A few grapes

1 small tin of peaches or pears in
    their own juice (not in syrup)

Method Combine all ingredients and serve with a slice of wholemeal toast and spread.

Baked Custard

1½ cups milk

1 tablespoon honey

2 eggs

Vanilla essence

Method Beat eggs and honey, add milk and vanilla essence. Pour into a pie dish lightly greased with coconut or olive oil. Cook gently, standing in a dish of water, until set. Serve with a round of wholemeal toast.

Scrambled Egg on Toast

1 large or 2 small eggs

½ teaspoon olive oil

1 tablespoon milk

Worcester sauce

2 slices wholemeal bread,

A little pepper and a pinch of sea

salt

Method Heat the olive oil in a small saucepan, blend in the beaten egg with the seasoning and Worcester sauce, stir well until scrambled. Toast the wholemeal bread and pile the scrambled egg on top.

Eggs with Mushroom Stuffing

¾ cup chopped mushrooms

2 teaspoons parsley

4 hard-boiled eggs (halved)

4 oz cottage cheese Worcester sauce

Olive or coconut oil

Method Fry the prepared chopped mushrooms with the parsley in a little olive or coconut oil. Remove the yolks from the hard-boiled eggs and mash them with the mushroom mixture, adding Worcester sauce and seasoning to taste. Fill the halved egg whites with the stuffing and place in a greased ovenproof dish. Cover with cottage cheese. Place under a pre-heated grill for 5–10 minutes.

Fluffy Egg Nests

2 eggs
2 slices hot wholemeal toast,
　drizzled with oil

Sea salt and pepper

Method First prepare the toast, then separate the eggs, leaving the yolks in the half-shells until required. Season the whites and beat them until stiff enough to form peaks. Pile the egg whites round the outer edges of the toast slices and drop the yolks into the centre. Season again. Place under a pre-heated grill and cook gently until the yolks are firm and the whites delicately tinged with brown. Serve on a hot dish and garnish with parsley. Serves two.

Grilled Mushrooms

Fresh mushrooms
Slices of wholemeal toast,
　drizzled with oil

Pepper and a little sea salt
Nutmeg

Method Wash the mushrooms, removing the skin and stalks. Brush with olive oil and sprinkle with sea salt, pepper and a little nutmeg. Place under a pre-heated grill, cap side up. Cook for 8–10 minutes. Serve on wholemeal toast.

Turkey Sausage on Toast

8 turkey sausages
Sunflower margarine

8 slices wholemeal bread, thinly
　cut

Method Grill the sausages. Remove the crusts from the bread, drizzle with olive oil on top side. Roll a sausage in each slice of bread, oil-side inwards. Place under the grill and toast evenly all round. This dish can be served with scrambled eggs or mushrooms.

Stuffed Turkey Sausages

10 turkey sausages
10 thin slices of lamb's liver
Egg, beaten
2 cups wholemeal breadcrumbs

1 small onion
A pinch each of sea salt and
   pepper
2 teaspoons sage

Method Mix together the crumbs, finely chopped onion, sage and seasoning and bind with egg. Split the sausages lengthwise and spread with the stuffing. Wrap each in a very thin slice of lamb's liver and secure with a cocktail stick. Place under a pre-heated grill and cook for approximately 10 minutes, turning as required. Serve at once.

Oats and Fruit Blend

¼ banana
1 teaspoon honey
2 dried apricots, soaked
   overnight in water

3½ oz bio/live yoghurt
2 oz oats, soaked overnight
   in water
1–2 teaspoons apple juice, to serve

Method Drain apricots and oats. Blend all ingredients together. Add a dash of apple juice.

Veggie Juice

2 stalks celery
1 cucumber
2 stalks fennel
½ inch root ginger, peeled
A handful of fresh leaves,
   e.g. lettuce, parsley, coriander,
   spinach, etc.

1 egg* (egg is used raw in this
   recipe, so choose the best quality,
   i.e. fresh, organic, free-range

Method Add celery, cucumber, fennel, ginger and leaves into juicer according to the instructions of your machine. Add raw egg and combine. *Protein powder (1 dessert spoonful) can be substituted for raw egg.

Fish dishes

Fish is a good source of nutrients; it is a protein food and provides omega-3 fatty acids. In the same way as varying meat intake, vary your intake of fish. Choose between white fish, oily fish and shellfish, with smoked fish rarely. They are all different in taste, texture and appearance.

- *White fish* – cod, grey mullet, gurnard, haddock, hake, halibut, lemon sole, plaice, red mullet, sea bass, sea bream, skate, turbot, whiting
- *Oily fish* – anchovies, eel, herring, kipper, mackerel, pilchards, salmon, sardines, sprats, swordfish, trout, tuna, whitebait
- *Shellfish* – crab, crayfish, langoustine, lobster, mussels, oysters, prawns, scallops, shrimp, squid.

Cod with Olives

1 lb fresh cod fillet	*1 egg*
1 tablespoon olive oil	*4–6 olives, halved*
Toasted crumbs (wholemeal)	

Method Prepare the cod by cleaning and cutting into small portions; coat with egg and then crumbs. Heat olive oil in frying pan over medium heat. Gently fry cod pieces, for 5–8 minutes, turning once. Garnish with olives and serve.

Grilled fish dishes

Sea Bass

1 whole sea bass, filleted	*Pepper*
Sunflower oil	*Parsley for garnish*
A pinch of sea salt	

Method Preheat grill. Brush both sides with a little oil. Cook under a pre-heated grill for about 8–10 minutes, turning once only. Season and serve garnished with parsley.

Grilled Haddock

1 medium-sized haddock

½ oz wholemeal flour

A little sea salt and pepper

Method Wash and trim the fish. Turn it in the seasoned flour. Place under a pre-heated grill and cook gently for 15 minutes, turning once. Serve on a hot dish garnished with parsley.

Grilled Salmon

Fresh salmon slices

Olive oil

Spring onions, chopped

Chopped parsley

1 or 2 anchovy fillets

Method Marinate the seasoned slices of salmon for about one hour in a mixture of olive oil, spring onions and parsley. Drain them well. Grill for approximately 8 minutes. Turn the slices over and cook for a further 5 minutes. Place the anchovy fillets on them and continue cooking for about 3 minutes. Serve with creamed potatoes and peas.

Oven fish dishes

Cod in Mushroom Sauce

4 cod steaks

1 tablespoon cider vinegar

FOR THE SAUCE

6 oz chopped mushrooms

4 tablespoons natural live yoghurt

2 oz cottage cheese

A little sea salt and pepper

Cucumber slices and parsley for garnish

Method Place the cod in an ovenproof dish and cover it with cider vinegar. Cook in the centre of a pre-heated oven, 180°C (350°F), gas mark 4, for 20–25 minutes. Mix all the sauce ingredients together and pour it over the cod steaks. Garnish with cucumber slices and parsley.

White Fish with Mushrooms

1 lb white fish fillet   ½ lb creamed potatoes
2 oz mushrooms   Parsley
Sea salt and pepper

FOR THE SAUCE
¼ pint fish stock or vegetable stock   ½ oz wholemeal flour
½ oz sunflower margarine

Method Prepare the fish and cut into small pieces. Place in a greased fireproof dish and sprinkle with a little sea salt and pepper. Add some of the chopped mushrooms. Cover the fish with stock. Bake in a moderate oven, 190°C (375°F), gas mark 5, for about 30 minutes. Strain off the liquid and use it to make a basic sauce with the fat and flour. Season to taste. Pipe creamed potatoes round the edge of the dish. Place under a hot grill for 10–15 minutes to brown the top. Serve garnished with parsley.

Plaice and Apple Bake

4 fillets of plaice, skinned   Parsley for garnish
1 tablespoon cider vinegar

FOR THE FILLING
1 small apple, peeled and sliced   4 oz cottage cheese
1 small green pepper, seeded and   A little black pepper
   halved

Method Chop half the apple and half the pepper (slice the remainder of each for garnish). Combine together all the filling ingredients.

Spread some on each of the fillets and roll them up. Place together in a casserole. Pour on the cider vinegar and cover. Cook in the centre of pre-heated oven, 190°C (375°F), gas mark 5, for approximately 30 minutes. Garnish with parsley and slices of pepper and apple. Serve with green beans and new potatoes.

Stuffed Trout with Almonds

4 medium-sized trout, cleaned and gutted

FOR THE STUFFING

1 tablespoon olive oil

1 small onion, peeled and finely chopped

4 oz wholemeal breadcrumbs

2 oz raisins

1 dessertspoon cider vinegar

2 sticks celery, chopped

2 tablespoons finely chopped parsley

3 tablespoons milk

2 oz flaked almonds

A little sea salt and freshly ground black pepper

Parsley for garnish

Method Wash the trout in cold water and wipe dry. Heat 1 tablespoon olive oil and sauté the onion until soft but not brown. Place the breadcrumbs, raisins, onion, cider vinegar, celery, parsley and almonds in a bowl and mix together thoroughly. Season and then fill the trout with this stuffing. Place the trout in an ovenproof dish. Pour milk over and sprinkle with flaked almonds. Cover with foil and bake in a pre-heated oven, 180°C (350°F), gas mark 4, for about 1 hour or, depending on the size of the trout, until the flesh is tender. Place on serving dish and garnish with parsley. Serve with boiled potatoes and a green vegetable.

Lunch dishes

Fish and Pasta Salad

12 oz smoked haddock, cooked,
  boned and flaked
4 oz packet frozen French beans,
  cooked according to instructions
6 oz pasta shells, cooked in boiling
  salted water for 13 minutes and
  drained

4 oz mushrooms, washed and
  sliced
2 tablespoons parsley

FOR THE DRESSING

4 tablespoons sunflower oil
2 tablespoons cider vinegar
½ teaspoon dry mustard

A pinch of demerara sugar
A little sea salt and pepper

Method Place all the dressing ingredients in a screw top jar and shake for a few seconds until thoroughly mixed. Mix together in a bowl all the salad ingredients and toss in the dressing.

Mackerel Pizza

FOR THE SCONE BASE

1 oz butter, melted
2 oz wholemeal flour
2 oz plain flour, sieved
½ teaspoon baking powder

½ teaspoon sea salt
½ teaspoon mixed herbs
1 egg, size 4
1 tablespoon milk

FOR THE TOPPING

1 tablespoon olive oil
1 onion, peeled and chopped
3 oz mushrooms, trimmed and
  chopped
7½ oz can mackerel, drained
  and flaked

A pinch of oregano
3 oz cottage cheese
Green olives, sliced, for garnish

Method Place all the ingredients for the scone base in a mixing bowl and use wooden spoon to mix. Turn on to a lightly floured surface and knead gently. Shape into a flat round, 8–9 inches in diameter, and place on a baking sheet. Heat oil and sauté onion and mushrooms. Add mackerel and oregano and spread over the scone base. Spread cottage cheese on top and garnish with olives. Bake in a hot oven, 200°C (400°F), gas mark 6, for 20–25 minutes. Serve hot or cold with a green salad.

Kipper Pâté

2 kippers
4 oz curd cheese
A pinch of cayenne pepper

A little sea salt and black pepper
1 tablespoon natural yoghurt

Method Poach kippers in water for 5–6 minutes and let them cool slightly in the liquid. Remove skin and bones. Place kipper flesh and remaining ingredients in a liquidizer and blend until smooth. Pile into a dish and serve with wholemeal toast spread with margarine.

Garlic Prawns

1 dessertspoon olive oil
6 large prawns (frozen prawns
    must be completely defrosted)

1 garlic clove, crushed
1 teaspoon fresh parsley, chopped

Method Heat the oil in a small frying pan. Add the garlic and prawns together. Gently heat the prawns through for 3–4 minutes (depending on size) and sprinkle on the parsley. Serve with salad leaves and wholemeal bread.

Meat dishes

When buying meat choose the leanest, and before cooking it trim off any visible fat; expensive cuts are not necessary. When browning meat and vegetables for casseroles, use olive oil, duck or goose fat.

Lamb Kebabs

12 oz leg lamb, boned, trimmed
  and cut into 1½ in cubes
4 oz button mushrooms
1 green pepper, de-seeded and cut
  into 1 in squares

8 bay leaves (optional)
Sunflower oil

Method Arrange lamb cubes, mushrooms, peppers and bay leaves on four long skewers. Brush with oil and place under a pre-heated grill for 10–12 minutes, turning and brushing regularly. Serve with boiled wholegrain rice and a mixed salad.

Lamb and Potato Curry

1 tablespoon olive oil
2 onions, finely chopped
1 clove garlic, crushed
1½ in piece of root ginger,
  peeled and chopped
1 teaspoon turmeric
1 tablespoon ground coriander
¼ teaspoon mild chilli powder
1 teaspoon ground cumin

1 tablespoon cardamom seeds,
  crushed
½ teaspoon ground cloves
2 lb lean lamb steaks, cubed
15 fl oz water
1 teaspoon sea salt
2 bay leaves
1 lb small potatoes, scrubbed

Method Heat oil in a large saucepan. Add the onions and garlic and fry until golden brown. Stir in the ginger, turmeric, coriander, chilli, cumin, cardamom and cloves. Fry for 4 minutes, stirring frequently. Add a spoonful or two of water, if the mixture becomes dry. Add the meat cubes and fry until evenly browned. Stir in the water, salt and bay leaves and bring to the boil. When the mixture begins to bubble, reduce the heat to a low simmer for 1¼ hours. Add the potatoes and bring to the boil again. Cover and simmer for another 45 minutes, or until the meat is cooked through and tender. Transfer the mixture to a warmed serving dish and serve at once. Makes four to six servings.

Lamb Kebabs

1 medium-sized onion, peeled and
    chopped
3 garlic cloves, crushed
1½ in piece of fresh root ginger,
    peeled and finely chopped
2 green chillis, finely chopped
2 tablespoons chopped coriander
    leaves
3 tablespoons natural yoghurt

½ teaspoon turmeric
1 tablespoon cider vinegar
1 teaspoon sea salt
½ oz fresh breadcrumbs
1½ lb minced lamb
2 tablespoons olive oil
1 oz melted sunflower margarine
Cucumber slices for garnish

Method Combine all the ingredients, except the cucumber, in a large bowl. Knead until the ingredients are blended and the mixture is stiff. Leave to stand for 30 minutes. Pre-heat the grill to high. Dip 12 skewers in oil. Dampen hands and remove small pieces of the meat mixture and shape them around the skewers. Put the skewers on a lined grill pan and drizzle with oil. Grill for 5 minutes. Turn over, drizzle with a little more oil and grill for another 5 minutes. Arrange the skewers on a bed of boiled wholegrain rice and garnish with slices of cucumber. Serve at once.

Braised Lamb with Peppers

1 tablespoon oil
2 lb shoulder lamb, boned and
    trimmed
1 large onion, sliced
1 large red pepper, de-seeded and
    sliced

½ pint stock
Pepper
6 oz potatoes, diced
8 oz frozen peas

Method Heat the oil in a large pan, add the lamb and brown it all over. Transfer the meat to a plate and add the onion and pepper to the pan. Stir fry until the vegetables begin to soften. Return the joint to the pan, placing it in the centre of the vegetables. Stir in the stock and seasoning and pour over the joint. Bring to the boil, cover pan and simmer for 1 hour. Add potatoes and peas, bring back to simmering point, replace the cover and continue cooking for a further 15 minutes. Transfer lamb to a warm serving dish and serve it sliced, with the vegetables and stock gravy. Serves four.

Lamb with Yoghurt Sauce

3 lamb steaks

3 tablespoons clear honey

3 tablespoons chopped mint

1 tablespoon cider vinegar

FOR THE SAUCE

½ pint natural yoghurt

1 tablespoon clear honey

1 tablespoon chopped parsley

1 tablespoon chopped mint

Method Place the meat in a dish. Mix together the mint, honey and cider vinegar, pour it over the meat and leave to marinate for 2 hours. Cook under a hot grill for approximately 10 minutes each side, basting occasionally with the marinade liquid. Mix the sauce ingredients together and serve with the meat. A green salad is excellent with this dish.

Lamb Steaks with Pepper

1 tablespoon olive oil

1 garlic clove, crushed

Sea salt and pepper to taste

1 lb lamb steaks, cut into strips

1 teaspoon soya sauce

2 teaspoons demerara sugar or
   honey

6 oz bean sprouts

2 green peppers, de-seeded and
   thinly sliced

½ tablespoon cornflour blended
   with 2 tablespoons water

4 spring onions, sliced

Method Heat oil in large frying pan. Add the garlic, salt and pepper and stir fry for 30 seconds. Add the lamb strips and stir fry for 3 minutes. Increase the heat to high. Stir in the soya sauce and sugar or honey and 2 tablespoons of water, cover and cook for 5 minutes. Uncover and stir in the bean sprouts and peppers. Cover again and simmer for 5 minutes. Stir in the cornflour until the mixture thickens. Put the mixture in a warmed serving dish, sprinkle it with spring onion and serve at once. Serves four.

Shepherd's Pie

1 lb lamb, minced
Olive oil
2 large carrots, chopped finely
1 large onion, chopped finely
1 clove garlic, crushed
2 + 1 teaspoons mixed herbs

1 level dessertspoon wholemeal
*   flour*
½ pint stock or water
1 lb potatoes, quartered
2 tablespoons milk
1 dessertspoon cheese, grated

Method In a large frying pan or saucepan, heat 1 tablespoon of olive oil. Add the carrots and onion. Cook over a medium heat for approximately 8 or 9 minutes, until browned at the edges. Add the lamb mince and increase the heat to brown quickly. Stir in the wholemeal flour. Add the stock or water, garlic and 2 teaspoons of mixed herbs and bring to boil. Reduce the heat to a gentle simmer and cook for 30 minutes. Meanwhile, in a separate pan, cook the potatoes in just enough water to cover them for 20 minutes. Drain and mash with 2 tablespoons of milk and 1 tablespoon of olive oil. Tip the lamb and vegetable mixture into an ovenproof dish and add the mashed potatoes on top, levelling them with a fork. Combine the grated cheese with 1 teaspoon of mixed herbs and place under a hot grill for 8–10 minutes to brown. Serve.

Lamb's Liver with Onions

2 dessertspoons olive oil
1 tablespoon wholemeal flour
1 onion, thinly sliced into rings

6 oz lamb's liver, cut into strips
Sea salt and pepper to taste
Chopped parsley

Method Heat the oil in a large frying pan. Add the onions, reduce heat to low and simmer, stirring occasionally, for 15 to 20 minutes, or until they are very soft. Meanwhile, put flour into a bowl and add salt and pepper. Coat strips of lamb's liver with the flour mixture. Add the strips to the pan, raise the heat to moderate, and fry them for 4–6 minutes, turning occasionally, or until they are cooked through and tender. Transfer the liver and onions to a warm serving dish and sprinkle with parsley. Serve at once.

Chicken dishes

Chicken with Tarragon

1 chicken, free-range   1 dessertspoon olive oil
1 bunch fresh tarragon

Method Pre-heat the oven to 190°C (375°F), gas mark 5. Place tarragon into cavity of chicken. Put the chicken into a roasting pan and drizzle with olive oil. Put the pan into the oven and roast the chicken for 30 minutes, then turn it over and roast for another 30 minutes. Reduce the oven temperature to moderate, 180°C (350°F), gas mark 4. Carefully turn the chicken again and continue to roast for a further 30 minutes, basting well, until the chicken is cooked through (the juices should run clear when you pierce the chicken with a skewer or fork). Remove from the oven and transfer the chicken to a warmed serving dish. Serve with new potatoes and vegetables. Serves six.

Spanish Chicken

¼ cup olive oil   2 cups chicken stock
4 lb chicken, cut into serving pieces   Sea salt and pepper to taste
2 medium onions, thinly sliced   ¼ teaspoon cayenne pepper
1 clove garlic, crushed   ½ teaspoon saffron threads soaked
1 large red pepper, de-seeded and   in tablespoon water
   chopped   16 olives, chopped
14 oz can artichoke hearts, drained

Method Pre-heat the oven to moderate, 180°C (350°F), gas mark 4. Heat the oil in a large, deep frying pan. Add the chicken pieces and fry until they are evenly browned. Using tongs, transfer the pieces as they brown to a large flameproof casserole. Add the onions, garlic and pepper to the pan and fry until they are soft. Add the artichoke hearts and fry for a further 2 minutes. Pour over the stock and stir in the seasoning, cayenne and saffron. Bring to the boil, stirring occasionally. Pour the mixture over the chicken pieces. Put the casserole in the oven and cook for 1 hour, or until the chicken pieces are cooked through and tender. Remove from the oven and transfer the chicken pieces to a warmed serving dish. Scatter with olives and serve.

Herbed Chicken Breasts

4 boneless chicken breasts
1 oz margarine
1 dessertspoon olive oil
3 oz flour

1 teaspoon fresh soft-leaf herbs
    such as basil, tarragon, parsley,
    coriander (or ½ teaspoon dried)
Sea salt and pepper

Method Pre-heat oven to 200°C (400°F), gas mark 6. Wash the chicken breasts and pat them dry with kitchen paper. Add the herbs to the flour and season with a small pinch of sea salt and pepper. Melt the margarine gently in a small pan and add the oil; remove from heat. Dip the chicken breasts into the margarine and oil mixture one by one, and place them into a food bag. Add the flour mixture to the bag. Hold the bag closed while inverting it and turning it around to completely coat the chicken breasts with the flour mixture. Place the chicken breasts on a baking tray and bake in the oven for 30 minutes or until cooked and golden.

Chicken and Nut Galantine

1 medium-sized roasting chicken
1 pint water
A pinch of sea salt
Freshly ground black pepper

4 oz chopped nuts
2 oz soft brown breadcrumbs
2 eggs, beaten
⅔ cup chicken stock

Method Cut all the flesh from the chicken and set aside. Put the bones and giblets in a saucepan with water and salt and pepper. Cover the pan and simmer for 1 hour. Mince the chicken with the meat from the giblets and add the nuts and breadcrumbs. Stir in the eggs and chicken stock and add salt and pepper to taste. Press the mixture into a well-greased 2 lb loaf tin and cover with greased foil. Stand in a roasting tin containing a little cold water. Place in a pre-heated moderate oven, 180°C (350°F), gas mark 4, and cook for 1–1½ hours. Leave to cool. Serve cold with salad or for picnics or packed lunches.

Normandy Chicken

2 tablespoons olive oil
3 lb chicken, cut into portions
2 shallots, finely chopped
1 oz wholemeal flour
2 cups cider vinegar
½ cup chicken stock

½ teaspoon dried sage
½ teaspoon dried thyme
Sea salt
Freshly ground black pepper
1 lb cooking apples, peeled, cored
    and thickly sliced

Method Heat the oil in a frying pan and fry the chicken portions until golden brown all over. Remove the chicken portions from the pan and transfer to a casserole. Fry the shallots in the fat remaining in the pan, then sprinkle in the flour and cook, stirring constantly, until light brown. Gradually stir in the cider vinegar, stock and herbs and bring to the boil, stirring constantly. Cook until the sauce has thickened, season to taste with sea salt and pepper and pour over the chicken. Cover the casserole, place in a pre-heated oven, 180°C (350°F), gas mark 4, and cook for 1 hour or until the chicken is just tender. Meanwhile put the apple slices into a pan and cook them for about 5 minutes, stirring occasionally until soft. Spoon the apples over the chicken, taste and adjust seasoning. Serves six.

Chicken with Mushroom Sauce

4 chicken pieces
½ teaspoon chopped fresh
    marjoram or rosemary
1 teaspoon sea salt
A pinch of freshly ground black
    pepper

1 teaspoon chopped fresh chives
2 tablespoons cider vinegar
¼ cup wholemeal flour
1¼ cups milk
1½ cups sliced mushrooms

Method Rub chicken pieces with olive oil. Put them into a deep casserole large enough to hold them. Sprinkle with herbs, salt and pepper, chives and cider vinegar. Cut the mushrooms into small pieces and add to chicken. Cover with foil or a lid. Place in a pre-heated oven, 180°C (350°F), gas mark 4, and bake for 45 minutes. Drain juices into a small saucepan, adding a little water if necessary, and stir in the flour. Cook, stirring, for 1 minute. Gradually add the milk, stirring continuously, and bring to the boil. Simmer for 2 minutes. Taste and adjust the seasoning. Serves four.

Chicken with Prunes

⅔ cup prunes, soaked
5 onions, 1 sliced and 4 quartered
1 bay leaf
6 peppercorns
1 cup cider vinegar
4 chicken pieces

4 tablespoons olive oil
¼ cup wholemeal flour
⅔ cup chicken stock
½ teaspoon sea salt
Freshly ground black pepper

Method Put the prunes in a saucepan with the sliced onion, bay leaf, peppercorns and cider vinegar. Bring slowly to the boil, then allow to cool. Add the chicken joints. Turn into a bowl, cover and leave to marinate overnight or for several hours in the refrigerator. Discard bay leaf. Strain off the marinade and set aside. Stone the prunes. Fry the chicken pieces quickly in oil until golden brown. Remove them from the pan. Blend the flour with the fat remaining in the pan and gradually return the marinade, stirring constantly. Bring to the boil, stirring. Add the stock, sea salt and pepper and stir well. Return the chicken, quartered onions and prunes to the pan. Cover and simmer for 45 minutes or until the chicken is tender. Taste and adjust the seasoning. Serves four.

Chicken and Mushroom Casserole

3 lb chicken, cut into pieces
2 tablespoons olive oil
¾ lb onions, peeled and
    chopped
4 celery stalks, cut into pieces
1 tablespoon wholemeal flour

1¼ pints chicken stock
1 bouquet garni
Sea salt
Freshly ground black pepper
1 cup button mushrooms

Method Fry the chicken in the margarine until golden brown all over, then transfer to casserole dish. Cook the onions and celery in the fat remaining in the pan for about 10 minutes, then stir in the flour and cook for 1 minute. Gradually add the stock and bring to the boil, stirring constantly. Add the bouquet garni, season with sea salt and pepper and pour the sauce over the chicken. Cover and place in a pre-heated moderate oven, 180°C (350°F), gas mark 4, and cook for 45 minutes. Add the mushrooms and cook for a further 15 minutes. Remove the bouquet garni. Taste and adjust the seasoning. Serve with boiled rice, peas and sweetcorn. Serves four.

Vegetarian recipes

Potato and Onion Omelette

Olive oil
½ teaspoon tamari
1 large open mushroom, chopped
1 large potato, diced

1 onion, chopped
2 eggs
Water
Pepper

Method Bring the diced potato to the boil in a small pan of water. Allow to simmer for 5 minutes, remove from heat and drain. Meanwhile, gently heat a tablespoon of olive oil in a non-stick frying pan, add the chopped onion and fry gently for 5 minutes or so until cooked and lightly browned. Add the chopped mushrooms. Sprinkle with tamari and stir for 2 minutes. Add the drained potato. Set aside. Break the eggs into a bowl and beat until thoroughly mixed. Add a small pinch of pepper and 1 tablespoon of water. Heat 1 teaspoon of olive oil in a clean omelette pan or small frying pan. When hot, pour in the eggs. Leave for about 1 minute over high heat to allow the bottom to set, then loosen the egg mixture from sides of pan and cook rapidly, tipping the pan from side to side so that the liquid egg flows underneath and cooks quickly. Before the egg is quite set, pour the potato, onion and mushroom mixture on to the centre of the omelette to gently reheat it for just 1 minute. Have a warm plate ready. When the egg has set to your liking, slip a palette knife or fish slice under the omelette and fold it away from the handle of the pan. Tip the omelette on to the warm plate and fold the last half carefully over on the top. Serve with green peas.

Mushroom and Cashew Nut Pilaff

½ cup brown rice
1 onion, sliced
Olive oil
1 garlic clove, crushed
2 celery sticks, sliced

4 cups button mushrooms, sliced
1 red pepper, sliced
1 green pepper, sliced
1 cup cashew nuts
½ teaspoon soy sauce, or tamari

Method Cook the rice according to the directions on the packet. Drain. Meanwhile, heat 1 tablespoon of olive oil in a pan and sauté the onion for 5 minutes. Add the garlic, celery, mushrooms, peppers and nuts. Mix together and fry for 2 minutes. Add the soy sauce or tamari to taste, fry for 2 more minutes. Add the cooked rice, mix together and heat through. Serves four.

Potato and Coriander Burgers

1½ lb potatoes, peeled and
  quartered
1/3 cup red lentils
½ teaspoon cumin seeds
2 tablespoons onion, finely
  chopped
3 tablespoons coriander, chopped

½ teaspoon ground coriander
Pinch of ground cumin
Pinch of cayenne pepper
Sea salt and freshly ground black
  pepper
Wholemeal flour for dusting
Olive oil

Method Boil the potatoes for 20 minutes. Mash. Boil the lentils in double their quantity of water (or according to packet directions) until soft. Drain thoroughly. Heat 2 tablespoons of olive oil and sauté the cumin seeds for a few seconds. Add the onion, coriander and spices, and stir for 2 minutes. Add the lentils, salt and pepper and simmer, stirring frequently, until the mixture is dry. Leave to cool. Divide the potatoes into 8 portions. Divide the lentil mix into 8 portions. Push a ball of lentil mix into each ball of potato. Press gently into a burger shape. Dust with flour, cover and chill until firm. Brush burgers with a little oil and grill, or fry, until golden brown on both sides. Serve with salad.

Dessert recipes

Apple Crumble

1 lb baking apples, peeled, cored and thinly sliced
½ cup Barbados sugar

FOR THE CRUMBLE TOPPING
5 oz rolled oats
1 oz walnuts, chopped
2 tablespoons demerara sugar
1 pinch ground ginger

1 pinch ground cinnamon
1½ dessertspoons nut butter,
  melted

Method Place the fruit in a pie dish, layering with sugar to taste. To make the topping add walnuts to oats, then mix together with the sugar, ginger, cinnamon and melted nut butter. Sprinkle the crumble evenly over the fruit, smooth the top and press down lightly. Place in a pre-heated oven, 210°C (425°F), gas mark 7, and bake for 20 minutes, then reduce the temperature to moderately hot, 190°C (375°F), gas mark 5, and cook for a further 45 minutes. Serves four.

Mixed Fruit Pudding

1 cup self-raising wholemeal flour
A pinch of sea salt
1 teaspoon baking powder
½ teaspoon mixed spice
½ teaspoon ground cinnamon
⅔ cup demerara sugar
2 cups fresh wholemeal
    breadcrumbs

⅓ cup raisins
½ cup currants
½ cup seedless white raisins
2 medium eggs, beaten
½ cup milk

Method Sift the flour, salt, baking powder, mixed spice and cinnamon together into a bowl and stir in the sugar, breadcrumbs and dried fruit. Stir in the beaten egg and enough milk to give a soft consistency. Spoon the mixture into a pudding basin rubbed with sunflower margarine. Cover with foil, making a pleat in the centre to allow for expansion. Secure the foil around the rim of the basin with string. Stand in a saucepan with boiling water to one-third the depth of the basin and steam for 2½ hours, topping up with boiling water when necessary. Serves four to six.

Almond and Brown Sugar Flan

FOR THE PASTRY
2 cups wholemeal flour
½ teaspoon sea salt

½ cup butter
1–2 tablespoons water

FOR THE FILLING
½ cup butter
⅔ cup demerara sugar
1 large egg, beaten
½ cup finely chopped, blanched
    almonds

1 cup self-raising wholemeal flour
    sifted with 1 teaspoon cinnamon
1 tablespoon milk
1 tablespoon seedless white raisins

Method To make the pastry, sift the flour and salt together into a bowl then rub in the butter until the mixture resembles fine bread-crumbs. Stir in enough water to make a firm dough. Knead the dough lightly on a floured surface for 1 minute. Wrap in foil and leave to chill in the refrigerator for 30 minutes. Roll out the dough on a floured surface and use to line an 8-inch flan tin. To make the filling, place the butter and sugar in a bowl and beat until the mixture is light and fluffy. Beat in the eggs and almonds a little at a time, then fold in the sifted flour and cinnamon alternately with the milk. Stir in the seedless white raisins and turn the mixture into the pastry-lined flan tin, smoothing the top with a knife. Place in a pre-heated, hot oven, 210°C (425°F), gas mark 7, and bake for 15 minutes, then reduce the temperature to moderate, 190°C (375°F), gas mark 5, and bake for a further 25 minutes or until browned. Remove the flan from the oven and leave to cool.

Cinnamon Apple Pancakes

FOR THE BATTER

1 cup wholemeal flour	*1 tablespoon corn oil*
A pinch of sea salt	*1¼ cups milk*
1 egg	*Olive oil for frying*

FOR THE FILLING

4 large baking apples, peeled, cored	*1 cup raw brown sugar*
and sliced	*½ cup water*
A pinch of ground cinnamon	

Method To make the batter, sift the flour and sea salt into a bowl. Blend in the egg, corn oil and enough milk to make a fairly thin batter. Heat a little oil in a frying pan. Drop 2 tablespoons of batter into the centre of the pan and tilt and rotate to spread it. Cook for 1 minute. Turn the pancake over and cook the other side for 1 minute. Turn the pancake out of the pan and make nine or ten more in the same way. Leave to cool. For the filling, put the apples, cinnamon, sugar and margarine in a saucepan and simmer gently for about 20 minutes or until the apple is tender, stirring occasion-ally. Roll some of the filling in each pancake and fry the pancake rolls in the margarine over moderate heat until they are golden brown all over. Pile on a warm serving dish and sprinkle with a mixture of sugar and cinnamon. Serve with soya or dairy-free ice cream. Serves five to six.

Apple and Almond Jelly

2 large, sweet eating apples
¼ lb ground almonds
¾ oz gelatine

½ pint water
½ pint apple juice
1 tablespoon thick honey

Method Grate the apples and mix with the almonds. Dissolve the gelatine in ½ pint of water and stir in the honey and apple juice. Put the apple mixture into a large mould and pour in the liquid. Allow to set, turn out and serve with soya or dairy-free ice cream.

Plain Sponge

¼ lb wholemeal flour, sieved
¼ lb brown sugar
3 oz butter

1 tablespoon milk
2 eggs

Method Cream the butter and sugar, add the eggs one at a time and beat thoroughly. Fold in the sieved flour. Add milk if necessary; the mixture should be fairly stiff. Divide into 7-inch sandwich tins and bake at 180°C (350°F), gas mark 4, for 15–20 minutes. Turn on to cake rack to cool or serve hot with custard made with skimmed or powdered milk.

For a healthy finish to a meal, I don't think there is anything to beat a fresh fruit salad. A variety of fruits such as melon, apple, banana, pear, apricot and peach (no citrus or any acid fruit) can be cut into small chunks and topped with a little dairy-free or soya ice cream.

6

Natural products

In recent years, there has been an upsurge in natural products for arthritis. Each of these products will, most likely, have helped some people with their arthritic symptoms – thank God that the research is being carried out and that the findings are being circulated to the general public. There is plenty of money available for the pharmaceutical companies to develop new drugs but precious little for companies and individuals trying to provide evidence, from their own discoveries, of the help that natural substances can give to arthritics. However, the cost of some of these products can be high, the claims made for them may be dubious, and the source of them may be strange; they may interact with other medications, and it may be unwise to take them if you have certain medical conditions. Before taking any natural remedy, it is wise to check that it is suitable for you specifically, first by asking your doctor. Your doctor may not know enough about the remedy to be able to advise you, so check with an appropriately trained practitioner such as a nutritional therapist, a herbalist or a homoeopathic practitioner.

If you have severe pain, it is tempting to take anything that might be able to help, despite these warnings. In this chapter, I shall endeavour to guide you as to whether the substance might be worth adding to the acid-removing programme described throughout this book. Should you decide to undertake this programme, some of the following substances are superfluous to requirements despite the fact that they may be very good supplements in themselves.

Women who are pregnant should not take supplements except under medical supervision. It is also very important to take advice if you have health problems such as diabetes, or if you are taking drug medications of any kind – for any health problem – since there may be interactions that are not addressed specifically below.

Alpha-lipoic acid

Alpha-lipoic acid is an antioxidant. There is no need to take it as an extra supplement. However, it is present in lamb's liver, which you should eat.

SAMe (S-adenosyl-methionine) ✗

SAMe is present in the body. It inactivates toxins and has an antidepressant effect as well as possessing anti-inflammatory, pain-relieving and tissue-healing properties. It is relatively new and there has been insufficient research to determine a safe dosage at this stage. I would not recommend its use as a supplement.

Ginger

Ginger root has anti-inflammatory and pain-relieving qualities. It is also helpful in the case of excess mucus. Supplements are not necessary, but ginger can be used in cooking, in ginger tea (steep a small piece of ginger root in boiling water for a few minutes, then drink the water), ginger biscuits and ginger cake – provided that beneficial ingredients are used (i.e. wholemeal flour, skimmed milk, molasses, etc.).

White willow bark ✓

This is an anti-inflammatory and pain-killing herb from which aspirin has been refined. The white willow bark is safer on the stomach than aspirin and can be very helpful for pain relief. It can be added to the Margaret Hills treatment.

Oils of cajeput (*Melaleuca leucodendron*), camphor, eucalyptus, fir needle, pine needle, rosemary   ✗

These are all oils that may relieve symptoms of arthritis. Before purchasing, check with a specialist practitioner who uses oils, such as an aromatherapist or massage therapist, that they are appropriate for you.

Capsaicin (Cayenne)

This is found in a cream, which may be applied for pain relief. It can also be used in cooking.

Boswellia serrata, cat's claw, devil's claw, horsetail, turmeric

These are all remedies with an anti-inflammatory action. It would be best to consult a herbalist before using them.

Mistletoe

Mistletoe injections – not mistletoe taken by mouth – have been found to alleviate inflammation around joints, but I would not recommend any such invasive procedures.

Glucosamine

Glucosamine is found naturally in the body. For supplements, it is normally manufactured from the shells of shellfish. It can be taken to help to relieve pain. Do not take it if you are allergic to iodine or shellfish. You should also not take it if you have blood sugar problems such as diabetes or hypoglycaemia.

Collagen

Collagen is extracted from the bones and skins of animals. Rather than taking it in supplement form, ensure you eat plenty of protein.

Chondroitin

Chondroitin is found naturally in the body. When it is manufactured, the source is generally from animals. It is often formulated with glucosamine. Check the source of chondroitin – most of it comes from bovine trachea (i.e. the windpipe of cattle), so ensure that it has been prepared from disease-free stock. An alternative source is shark cartilage, which tends to be more expensive.

Copper

Rheumatoid arthritis sufferers can be deficient in copper. However, because copper is present in recommended foods such as honey, molasses, lentils and mushrooms, it is probably unnecessary to take it as a food supplement. Diabetics who cannot take honey or molasses may benefit from a small regular intake. Copper bracelets may be worn.

Garlic, lycopene, glucosinalates, catechins and quercetin

These plants and plant extracts are good antioxidants that help to neutralize toxins. There is normally no need for a supplement, but you should include broccoli, garlic, onions, apples and green tea in your diet, since these foods are excellent sources of these antioxidants.

Boron

Boron is a mineral that has a good effect on calcium metabolism. There is no need to take it in supplement form provided you take alfalfa and kelp, which are good sources of boron. Also eat cabbage and leafy greens for their boron content.

MSM (methyl-sulfonyl methane)

MSM is manufactured in the body from sulphur-containing amino acids. There is no need to take it as a supplement provided you eat skimmed milk, fish, fresh vegetables and also take soya protein isolate powder daily, such as found in the 'Margaret Hills Protein'.

Sulphur

See MSM.

Zinc

Zinc is vital for many enzymatic functions in the body. Most arthritics are deficient in this mineral. It is useful as a supplement when taken with other minerals and vitamins, but it should not be taken continuously for an extended period without supervision.

Green-lipped mussel

Green-lipped mussel has pain-relieving and anti-inflammatory properties, but there is no need for it in supplement form if you eat fish and, occasionally, shellfish.

Reishi mushroom

This has been used in China for thousands of years to relieve symptoms of arthritis among other problems. There is no need to take it as a supplement but you can include dried and fresh mushrooms in your diet. Dried mushrooms add an intense flavour so only a little should be added to any fresh mushroom dish.

DLPA (DL-phenylalanine)

DLPA can reduce chronic pain by inhibiting an enzyme that breaks down the body's natural painkillers. It can be very useful for pain relief in supplement form but not if you have high blood pressure or are taking certain medications – so seek advice.

SOD (superoxide dismutase)

The body produces this antioxidant, and there is no need to take it as a supplement. It occurs in food – ensure that you eat broccoli, brussels sprouts, cabbage, other green vegetables and wheat.

DMSO (dimethyl sulfoxide)

DMSO is a waste product of the paper-making industry, and it has been used as a commercial solvent. It is claimed that it was the first non-steroidal anti-inflammatory drug to be discovered. However, side-effects include an odour emanating from the patient and the possibility of headaches. As with any pharmaceutical agent, it is not recommended.

CMO (cerasomal-cis-9-cetylmyristoleate)

CMO is a beef by-product (bovine tallow), which acts as an anti-inflammatory agent. Beef and beef products should be avoided when following the acid-removing programme for arthritis.

DHEA (dehydroepiandrosterone)

DHEA is a controversial hormone available in supplement form. It is easily converted into other hormones, especially oestrogen and testosterone. I do not recommend its use.

Betaine, bromelain, papain, pepsin, trypsin, rennin, pancreatin and chymotrypsin

These are all enzymes that aid digestion and also help with anti-inflammatory activity. There is no need to take them in supplement form because cider vinegar covers this function, as does honey.

The most effective way to combat arthritis is to follow the pro-gramme given in this book – an acid-free diet, the acid-removing treatment with cider vinegar drinks, molasses and Epsom salts baths, and appropriate nutritional supplements. You are welcome to contact the Clinic for personal advice if necessary. This can be invaluable if you have other health problems or are taking drug medication for any reason.

There are rarely effective short cuts for the relief of arthritis that have a long-term benefit. A great deal of time and money can be invested in trying the above supplements when the simple straight-forward approach is far more effective and beneficial to your overall health and well-being.

7

The Clinic

Positive thinking is the essence of all healing. Many patients have said to me that they came to my Clinic full of miseries – and went away full of hope. Hopeful that they are going to feel better in a short time and hopeful that eventually they will get rid of their arthritis. Faith in oneself is the essence of joyful living – when one has faith, there is no room for worry. Worry is the downfall of all who can't fight it – so I say, don't try to fight it. Instead adopt a positive mental attitude and when waking each morning, thank God for allowing you to wake up, and for giving you the opportunity to enjoy the beautiful new day that he has ordained for you, think of other people and how you can help them, and it's surprising the sense of well-being and satisfaction that one derives from a kind thought, word or deed, projected in the direction of others.

Always think pleasant and happy thoughts as you lay your head on your pillow, because you shape and build your character and willpower while you are asleep. If your dominant thought when you fall asleep is cheerful and happy, you will wake up cheerful, strong and resolute to begin another day. Always aim high and don't be content with pettiness, and above all watch a 'don't care' frame of mind. Forget the past, that is gone – look to a bright, happy and successful future. It is what you are capable of doing now that matters, and you are capable of big things if you will put your shoulder to the wheel and push with all your might.

Don't fear, don't fret, don't anticipate evil, don't fear anything for there is nothing to fear, fret or worry about. Hold your head high, look the world in the face, fight the good fight and victory will be yours.

I find that most people that I see at the Clinic think negatively, and I am fully convinced that this negative thinking destroys them. 'There is no cure – you must learn to live with it' – what negative thinking, and what a death sentence! That sentence was pronounced on me, and to this day I believe that if I didn't have a husband and a large family to look after, I might not have had the willpower to fight the good fight and rid myself of that painful body that was the result of wrong diet. However, I thank the Lord that he gave me so many reasons to explore every channel for the promotion of good health, and a pain-free busy life.

Previous editions of this book have now travelled far and wide; the message within them has been explored by thousands of people, most of whom we have never seen. We sometimes hear about them though.

In December 2002, Eileen from New Hampshire in the USA wrote on the Amazon website:

> I was given this book at 18 years of age. I had been suffering from RA for the previous seven years. At that point in my life, I thought everything was hopeless: I'd never be able to work; no one would ever want to marry me; and I would end up alone and in pain for the rest of my life. Needless to say – none of this happened. This book changed my life. At 18, I put heart and soul into following the recommendations. Within a couple of weeks, I went off my meds (much to my MD's disapproval, mind you!) and have not looked back since. I have not had a flare up in 15 years (I am now 33) . . .

A common experience for many is negativity from the medical profession, the members of which are trained in the power of pharmaceutical drugs but have little training in the power of good nutrition. However, as individual doctors witness improvement from patients determined to follow a drug-free path, they are gradually accepting that there might be a better way forward for some of their patients.

In 2007, Nancy wrote to me:

> This is to tell you that I have decided to give up the medication that you have been supplying for many years and from which I have benefited so much, and to see how I get on 'going it alone'. I would also like to thank you so very much for all you have done for me, and for letting me carry on a normal and very active life without being harassed by nagging pain. Without your help, I know I would not have been able to do half the things I have done and I feel truly grateful. I shall carry on with the diet

. . . I would also like to thank you for coming to my aid when I was suffering dreadful stomach troubles and for supplying me with the 'magic' potion which cured a problem which had been tormenting me for years. My daughter, who is a GP, has recommended you to some of her patients as she saw how much I was benefiting from your diet.

This is how the word spreads . . .

From the age of 16, Caroline, a 46-year-old widow with a 13-year-old son, had battled with arthritis and iritis, for which she had been hospitalized twice. When she contacted the Clinic in September 2001, she had been bedbound for several weeks with acute arthritis, mainly in her knees, feet and hands, and, from time to time, in her neck, shoulders and hips. She was taking meloxicam and pantaprazole. By April 2002, she had stopped taking her drugs and was describing her symptoms as mild, although her joints sounded like firecrackers going off when she moved. With no arthritic symptoms from October 2002 onwards, she wrote in April 2003 to say: 'I am completely free of pain; during the treatment I felt supported and had renewed hope and faith that the natural approach would help.' So much is down to one's own determination and belief.

Don, aged 84, approached the Clinic in March 2000. He was taking four types of medication following a stroke 15 years earlier. He was suffering with depression and arthritis. I created a treatment programme that would not interfere with his medication. Just five months later he was free of arthritis, with no pain at all. He commented: 'I feel so well and full of life.' What a marvellous feeling to have at the age of 84.

Bryan was struggling with arthritis pain in his shoulders and ankles when he contacted the Clinic in 2001. He had been experiencing pain in his lower spine and knees, which he thought might be due to playing squash for 40 years. In less than one year, this 67-year-old man reported being completely free from pain.

Alexandra, aged 50, was a very busy medical secretary, much of whose work involved using a computer keyboard. The pain and swelling in her wrists, elbows and shoulder were affecting her ability to work despite the anti-inflammatory drug she took. She suffered pain in her wrists, elbows, shoulder, hip, ankles, feet and knees, and she had breast pain. In 1999, she adopted a diet and supplement programme suitable for her vegetarian lifestyle. By September 2002, all her symptoms had disappeared and her joints were much improved.

Connie, a woman of 75, had always had good health until her right knee swelled up and she couldn't put any weight on it at all. Her left knee also began to cause her pain. Her doctor diagnosed arthritis. In November 2001, she started her treatment programme. Fourteen months later she wrote to say:

> This time last year I could hardly bear to put my foot down because of the pain – I was hobbling about – but now I am walking normally. Last Sunday, I did an eight-mile walk in snow over hills in the Dales, so that can't be bad! I must say I feel better in myself but it takes a lot of willpower, and you must really be determined to get better.

Such determination has its own rewards; it is hugely satisfying to find health and mobility improving as age creeps on, rather than the opposite.

Sister Frances also suffered from arthritis of the knee. She was in much pain and unable to walk properly. It is not an easy matter to follow a special diet when living in a community. She did her best and wrote:

> I persevered with the treatment for nearly three years. Now I am free from pain and I am able to walk normally. It has given me a new lease of life as some other minor ailments that I had have also been healed. I would wholeheartedly recommend it to anyone.

In 2008, Judy wrote:

> I was diagnosed as having arthritis in 1960 and was told both knees and hips would need replacing; my joints were stiff and painful, also walking any distance was quite difficult. Thirteen years ago, I discovered Margaret Hills' books and decided to try out the diet; within six months I felt so much better, pain and stiffness decreasing all the time. Taking the formula and protein made a great difference to my health and outlook, and all symptoms and pain had just about gone when, in 2004, I was diagnosed with polymyalgia rheumatica. Christine Horner told me that this illness came under the same umbrella as arthritis, and the diet, etc., would help – which it did. By 2007, I was

given a clean bill of health without taking any medication at all, instead of the possibility of having it for life. I am so thankful that I found the Margaret Hills Clinic, and for all the help and advice received over the years.

My patients become my friends; I take a personal interest in each and every one of them. To treat a patient properly one has to ascertain an overall picture of the patient's lifestyle, his or her worries and frustrations, because these play an important part in the attitude of a patient towards the illness.

As Margaret wrote in 2010:

> I'm so grateful for all you've done for me. I consider it a privilege to have come to the Clinic. I feel as though we're part of the family and, in this respect, I'm sorry I'm not coming anymore. I'm . . . spring cleaning and painting the pantry and all the woodwork throughout the house, plus decorating the lounge and kitchen. I feel on top of the world, so I think now is the time to stop coming to the Clinic . . . Much love, Margaret.

Very often a patient will come to my Clinic, having lost a spouse recently; he will tell me he is living alone and trying to adjust to life without his partner. He says his arthritis has got much worse since his partner passed away. He can see himself ending up in a wheelchair with nobody to look after him, and he projects a picture of hopelessness. I try to tell this patient that there is nothing to fear in life except fear. I ask him to cast out fear and look forward with hope; not just a vague hope in the mind, but hope throbbing as a life force in the heart. I say that death does not divide, there is no need to fear separation and death can never separate souls who love. It is very comforting to realize that however difficult you find life, if you accept your circumstances graciously and thankfully you will press forward rekindled by the fires of hope and know that in the end all will be well.

Usually when somebody falls sick something is lacking, and there is an imbalance in the patient's soul. Sometimes it is very difficult to ascertain the reasons for that imbalance; sometimes it is never ascertained, but with most people, as I gain their confidence, little by little the story unfolds and gradually I can see the reason, or reasons, for their state of ill-health.

I believe in helping my patients to help themselves, and as every healer knows, true healing begins with the spirit. As soon as the spirit practises pure thinking, pure living and pure action, it experiences a sense of well-being not previously known and starts to live harmoniously within itself. The aches, pains and frustrations recede into the background and a sense of faith in himself, coupled with a hopeful attitude, and kindness towards his fellow man replaces them. The power of positive thinking can bring forth beauty and harmony in a patient's life and by good, constructive ideas he can help to bring about that which is desirable and good.

Quite often I receive letters or phone calls of gratitude from my patients; it is encouraging to me to know that yet another of my patients is free of pain and does not require my services any longer. I give thanks to God and feel very humble and grateful that I have once again been instrumental in relieving another's pain and enabling that person to lead a pain-free, balanced, useful life. The number of people who follow the directions without needing help from the Clinic is impossible to determine. For example, a 2007 Amazon website review of a previous edition of this book mentions a 19-year-old with juvenile arthritis. It reads:

> He had been told he would be in a wheelchair in a few years, and he would never walk properly again. He was taking eight ibuprofen a day at the time, and still couldn't walk more than a few meters. He is now 100 per cent recovered, has taken NO medication from the doctors (he refused, based on the horrendous side-effects) and, as I write this, he is back at work as a plasterer. The doctor . . . is now very interested indeed! He has been discharged from hospital, and he officially doesn't have juvenile arthritis any more!

Another review on the Amazon website suggests that improvement is on the way for Bethany, who also has juvenile arthritis. It reads:

> We had been told time and time again that Bethany's diet would not in any way make her juvenile arthritis worse. However, after reading your plan and realizing that, although I thought I was giving her a healthy diet, she was having a lot of citrus foods. We have been following [your recommendations] for four days and we are seeing an improvement already. Having a young child on

so many drugs and injections is a real worry and if this will help even a bit, it will be the answer to all our prayers.

Perhaps the following extract from a patient's letter to Margaret Hills will encourage the reader not to lose heart and set about self-help, as this patient has done:

> I am filled with gratitude for the help you gave me, getting me to walk like a human being again. What a wreck I was, crying, cringing, a mess of a woman, in complete despair – you changed all that. I stuck to your diet and treatment religiously: now, here I am, decorating the house, and gardening and trimming my poodle. I am back in the stream of life, not 'up the creek' as I surely thought I was.

The above patient was brought to my Clinic on 18 June 1983. She could not sit on a chair and had been lying on her back for five months, under medical care. She had to lie on the floor on an eiderdown while I examined her. She had lost a lot of weight and was very confused. I knelt on the floor beside her and put my hands on her back asking if that was where the trouble was. She said, 'Yes, that's it. Please keep your hands there, don't take them away, they are very hot.' I realized that my hands were being used to bring warmth and comfort to the patient and I prayed that the pain would go. When I stood up after 15 minutes, the pain had gone and the patient stood up straight for the first time in five months and cried tears of joy, saying 'I'm healed'. She walked out to the car. I phoned her on Monday, 20 June at 9 a.m. to confirm the healing: she reported that she had been feeling fantastic since Saturday. She had made early morning tea and hoovered through the house. For the past 11 months she has followed the treatment and diet I set out for her; now she has put on weight and is doing all the things she wants to do – or as she puts it, she is 'back in the stream of life'. I do not profess to be a spiritual healer, although I do believe wholeheartedly in spiritual healing – but something happened that Saturday afternoon in June 1983 that both my patient and I will never cease to give thanks for.

On 12 June 1982 an article appeared in the *Coventry Evening*

Telegraph. It read as follows: 'Nobody knows what causes arthritis, there is no cure for it, the Coventry Council are spending X amounts of money on research and in three years they hope to come up with a cure.' Needless to say, they are now thirty years on and they still haven't found a cure and probably never will while they look to drugs for the answer. The cure lies in our own efforts to rid our bodies of excess acid, to keep to an acid-free diet and partake of the vitamins and minerals necessary to return to a state of health.

I hope and pray that this book will help to alleviate at least some of the pain and suffering, and bring hope to so many who have heard those hopeless words 'there is no cure – you must learn to live with it'. I say, be hopeful; now you know there is a cure and you do not have to learn to live with it, but remember, perseverance is the answer.

Some words from Jennifer, a diabetic, aged 68:

I am writing to thank you for your help in treating my arthritis, which has virtually disappeared, and to express my gratitude. At the start of September 2005, my doctor diagnosed arthritis in my neck. I was having pain and discomfort in it – there was not a full range of movement – and I found it almost impossible to sit comfortably on our sofa. Having been given some cream and exercises, and told there wasn't really anything that could bring about any improvement in it, I went away feeling rather depressed. The effect of the cream only lasted about a week, so I then tried taking glucosamine and chondroitin for a few months, during which time the condition remained static. Suddenly my neck got much worse. It kept 'seizing up' and 'locking'. The only relief was to put a heat pad on as soon as possible and to use a 'neck cushion'. The way things were going really frightened me, and then someone lent me your book. After reading it, I immediately filled in the questionnaire form* and became a postal patient, starting in April 2006. From that time on, there was a gradual improvement in my neck. It doesn't happen all at once – you have to stick at it for the long term. I found that the 'seizing up' had stopped, and gradually I was becoming less conscious of my neck with every passing day. I now have a complete range

---

*Go to <www.margarethillsclinic.com> for the questionnaire or contact the Clinic.

of movement, can sit comfortably, and actually forget about it. I have been able to take up playing table tennis again, which I love, and people have no idea that I ever had any problems with my neck at all. When I look back at how I was and the difference there is today, I am still amazed and so thankful. This treatment works; I have no hesitation in recommending it to anyone suffering from arthritis. Your books, in my opinion, should be read by all doctors everywhere.

I hope that by now the reader will have adopted a positive attitude of mind towards his or her illness and I should like everyone to remember the old adage – 'Whatever the mind of man can believe and perceive, it can achieve.'

I thank you for reading this book and hope you will benefit from it. May I also thank my many patients who have helped me and taught me so much along the way.

Good luck and God bless you all.

Appendix 1
Troubleshooting – overcoming
barriers to success

Since every person is different in his or her response to the Margaret Hills programme for arthritis, we'd like to highlight some of the potential barriers to improvement. After being on the programme for several months, it is sometimes the case that people find they are not as well as they thought they would be at this stage. This is the time when a Clinic consultation (either in person or on the phone) is vital to discover any obstacles that may be in the way of success.

This appendix is designed to illustrate that no two cases of arthritis are the same. The most important point to remember is that you are being helped as a whole person; the programme is not designed to treat your symptoms in isolation.

Other health conditions

Problems with your joints can be considered to be arthritis when in fact an underlying cause may have been missed. Doctors and consultants generally go to great lengths to eliminate other possible causes before diagnosing an arthritic condition, so if you have not actually received a diagnosis, do consult your GP and let us know the outcome.

Joint pains and inflammation can be the result of other conditions, such as hypothyroidism. A nurse from Ruislip with thyrotoxicosis wrote after six months on the treatment:

> I feel so much better. The awful depression has gone, and the pain in my knees and ankles has eased so much. I still have some pain at night. I have dropped all my medication. There's a light at the end of the tunnel and it's getting nearer and nearer. When I look back to last April, I could see no end to the awful pain. My family and friends are noticing the change.

Joint and muscle pains may be caused by many common drugs.

The solution

1 Contact us at the Clinic so we can assess your individual case and try to ascertain the reasons for lack of improvement.
2 Give as much detail as possible when registering as a patient of the Clinic. Include information about all prescribed medications you take, whether for arthritis or not, not forgetting hormone treatment such as the contraceptive pill or hormone replacement therapy. Include any 'over-the-counter' remedies you purchase routinely from the chemist or pharmacy. Also include any creams or gels that you apply – whether for pain relief or for any other condition.
3 If you have other health concerns, whether diagnosed or not – for example, frequent headaches or constipation, thyroid dysfunction, psoriasis or asthma – include them when registering or, if you forget, let us know when you remember. We can then investigate further and tailor treatment to be specific to you from the outset so your progress is much better.

Stress!

'Stress' is a word that is used frequently to describe how we are feeling but if left or dismissed this can have such a negative impact on our health. More often than not, patients report that their arthritis onset was triggered by a stressful event such as a divorce or a house move. Emotional difficulties are underlying so many health problems including arthritis, and unless they are addressed your recovery will be very much impaired. Stress is such an important factor in your overall well-being that a whole book could be written just on its effects. It increases the levels of inflammation in your body and increases your body's requirements for nutrients just to keep going.

When you have been diagnosed with an arthritic disease, fear can influence whether you improve or worsen as time goes on. Negative attitudes are unhelpful but it is natural to worry, especially when you are suffering with pain and discomfort. It is, however, incredibly important to address the fear and put it behind you. We can help you do this.

Nowadays, men, women and children face different challenges from those of yesteryear. For example, messaging via mobile phone, email, texts, voicemail – the speed at which we can communicate seems to require a fast response. Constant contact throughout the day is an interruption to the concentration necessary to complete the job at hand, making tasks take longer than necessary, so lengthening the working day and causing frustration. The more it happens, the more stressful it becomes. Add in lengthy travel to and from work, long hours, deadlines, etc., and it is easy to see the stress accumulating day by day.

Children and young people often nowadays find themselves living apart from one of their parents and have decisions to make regarding contact with them. This can be disruptive to hobbies and friendships. There has always been peer pressure but recent challenges include pressure to take recreational drugs and have sexual relationships. Youngsters have to be strong to resist such pressures and can succumb despite their good intentions, leading to feelings of inadequacy and regret.

The solution

Contact the Clinic if you feel that stress or emotional difficulties are bothering you. This may be an appropriate time to have a consultation, whether in person or on the telephone, dependent on where you live and how mobile you are. At this appointment, we can evaluate the extent to which your emotional health is hampering your recovery and discuss what steps can be taken to alleviate or remedy the situation. Your fears and worries can be addressed openly and in confidence in order to promote a positive attitude.

In terms of emotional upheaval, our specialism is in nutritional support for helping you to get through it. Various laboratory tests at our disposal look into the effect that stress has had on your body and can help us provide the nutritional solution for building your strength back up again. Addressing the stress is often necessary before the symptoms of arthritis clear from your body totally.

Digestive health

You have probably heard the saying that good digestion is the key to good health. This is *truer* than you can imagine. The digestive tract is where all nutrients from food are absorbed into the bloodstream. It is also where we have a high proportion of our immune system defences, such as lymphoid tissue (groups of cells which protect the body from bacteria and other foreign substances). Lymphoid tissue is in the tonsils, adenoids, oesophagus, stomach, intestines and appendix. For example, mucus and saliva contain enzymes and antibodies necessary for neutralizing microorganisms; stomach cells produce acid to kill micro-organisms that enter along with food; and friendly bacteria within the intestinal tract inhibit unhealthy bacteria overgrowth. The digestive tract is additionally where toxins and waste products are isolated and excreted. So problems in any part of the digestive system will affect your health and, consequently, your recovery from arthritis.

Phyllis is a typical example of how problems in the digestive tract can affect the whole body. She had pain and swelling in her joints when she contacted us in October 2009. She also suffered with severe fatigue, bloating and wind, felt drowsy, uncoordinated, dizzy and 'spacy'. She had constant pain beneath her ribcage and had difficulties eating. We addressed these problems by asking Phyllis to avoid specific foods and take certain nutritional supplements to support digestive health. Three months later Phyllis reported: 'I am delighted to report that my health is almost back to normal and my B12 levels have risen . . . as part of this, I seem to have lost any trace of food intolerances.'

The solution

If you have any recurring symptoms, please inform the Clinic so we can assess whether any further action is needed. These symptoms may include, for example, constipation, diarrhoea, loose stools, bloating, pain in your abdomen, acid reflux, indigestion, food intolerances, food allergies, heartburn, tiredness after eating, irritability or shakiness if hungry, recurrent thrush, urinary tract infections, and many more.

Frequent comments

In our view, a person develops an arthritic disease because his or her body has become too acidic. Many factors are involved in this accumulation of acid. We need to take into account anything and everything that may have led to the development of arthritis, i.e. all health conditions, the possible consequences from taking prescribed medications, dietary and lifestyle influences, and so on. Our overall aim is to help you vastly improve all aspects of your health and recover good mobility and a feeling of well-being. We address the same issues repeatedly when talking to patients and so here are some typical questions that we are frequently asked, with our responses.

'I don't need you to take care of my blood pressure – this is controlled by medication'

It is not possible to achieve complete success by ignoring other health factors. If your blood pressure is well controlled by medication this is fine, although the nature of our work is to delve deeper to discover why your blood pressure has risen in the first place. In other words, we look for the underlying cause – which also gives clues about how you may have acquired joint problems.

'It is my age; I'm not expecting to get any better, only worse as I get older'

You must have the goal in mind of returning to your former, active, healthy self. We have had people approach us for help when they are in their late 90s because they are not yet ready to give up. In fact, our oldest patient to date was 103 when she started; she improved greatly so that she was still able to fly to visit her family abroad. Such people do improve and have a much better quality of life. If you are only in your 60s or 70s or younger with arthritis, and 'put it all down to age' then you must try to think positively as you need to get rid of these symptoms as early as you can. Margaret Hills had very severe arthritis – both osteo- and rheumatoid – and managed to recover; even till her last days she never had any recurrence of her arthritis.

There is a 'wear and tear' issue with the onset of osteoarthritis but this too can be helped; we look at removing the factors that are putting this extra strain on your body. Ageing isn't a process of your body slowly falling apart; science now understands the metabolic factors behind ageing and so we, as nutritional medicine practitioners, can work with that and use supplements accordingly. The right supplements can make an incredible difference to your life.

For inspiration, you can perhaps take a photo of yourself dancing or doing something that was special – an activity or hobby you did before being stopped in your tracks by arthritis. You *can* regain your former self. It is so satisfying when you do, because you have not only got rid of the pain and other symptoms but you are also a much healthier, happier person, able to go on living your life in a much better way.

'I'm too young to get arthritis'

How young is young? Many young people and children get arthritis. Joint pains and inflammation are now common complaints among people in their 20s and 30s. Mothers can unwittingly pass on excess acidity to their newborn babies, which manifests as arthritis from a very young age. If you are under 18 years old it is essential that you attend for a consultation in person as we have to see you to be able effectively to advise you.

The modern average diet is responsible to some degree for many ill-health symptoms, including arthritis. With many people not having even the most basic cooking skills and preferring to put a 'ready meal' in the microwave, these problems are ever-increasing. The importance of food is so understated in our current times. Apart from obvious effects such as obesity, so many illnesses such as cancer, diabetes, cardiovascular disease, etc., are on the rise because it is not common knowledge how actually to eat well. Even healthy-eating sections in the supermarket can often get it wrong, by using artificial chemicals, sweeteners, preservatives and so on instead of just promoting pure, fresh, recognizable foods. It is no surprise that such illnesses are affecting so many people.

'It's my immune system attacking my joints so it won't work for me'

Autoimmune disease is responsible for certain types of arthritis. We look at the reasons why your immune system is responding in this way and advise accordingly. Here are some examples:

1 Medications taken for excess acid, ulcers, reflux, dyspepsia or indigestion can interfere with the body's immune system.
2 If the major detoxification organs such as the liver, kidneys, colon, lungs and skin are overloaded, toxins cannot be easily eliminated. Such toxicity sets the scene for autoimmune disease.
3 Drugs that inhibit inflammation may help reduce pain but in doing so they can weaken the immune system.
4 Infection sometimes precedes the onset of autoimmune disease; the immune system was already impaired to some degree in order to succumb to the infection.

The underlying causes need to be addressed; if you are not making much progress don't hesitate to get in touch at the Clinic, where we will consider how best to intervene.

'I have been following the directions in the book and feel much better but now I seem to have come to a standstill. Why is this?'

This is very often the case, as many people like to give things a go before really committing themselves. It is of the utmost importance to follow all the aspects of the treatment together, as this is how you achieve the full benefits. This includes the three main aspects:

1 removing the acid build-up from your body and encouraging better acid–alkaline balance;
2 avoiding the intake of acidic foods and increasing the intake of alkalizing foods;
3 replenishing your body's nutrients in the form of nutritional supplements. This is essential as your requirements for certain nutrients are greatly increased when the body is trying to overcome illness or disease.

Register with us at the Clinic; the fee is minimal and we do recommend it because we can then offer you our expertise in getting you well again. It is not enough to just drink cider vinegar and try to stick to the diet. Improvement is inhibited unless the right supplements are taken. However, you might be doing everything in exactly the right way but need a boost of energy to be able to instigate change. This is when a visit could be of benefit because you could have a treatment session that makes use of the Scenar, the InterX, a low-level laser or a therapeutic blanket. These relaxing treatments increase energy in the body and gently remind your brain that healing is required, often triggering an improvement in symptoms.

'I already take supplements so I don't need any more'

It might be that you are taking the wrong products in a poor-quality form or in the wrong dosage or combination. Many people take supplements that do not actually help the underlying problem. We guide you to taking the right supplements in order to achieve maximum absorption, assimilation and utilization by your body.

'I have a good diet so I don't think I need supplements'

Whenever there is a health problem, the right supplements can make a difference between improvement and further deterioration. The good diet that you think you have may, in fact, have contributed to the accumulation of excess acidity. If you keep a food diary over a period of two weeks and pass it on to us when you register, we can determine whether it would be wise to make changes.

Remember that a lack of exercise is often a consequence of arthritis. As arthritis progresses, it prevents the usual game of golf or evening of dancing, as well as inhibiting the duration and speed of walking. Nutritional supplements play an important role in improving the function and strength of both muscles and joints affected.

Additionally, certain drugs deplete nutrients from your body, or affect the action of nutrients. If you take medication for any reason, you would benefit from taking appropriate nutritional supplements. For example, NSAIDs (anti-inflammatory drugs) reduce iron levels in the blood and cause retention of sodium; steroids interfere with activation of vitamin D and decrease blood levels of magnesium, potassium, zinc, and vitamins A, B6, C and K; some blood-pressure medications cause decreased blood levels of zinc; some antacids cause decreased absorption of folic acid and copper; antibiotics decrease absorption of all nutrients; cholesterol-lowering drugs cause decreased blood levels of CoQ10; diabetic medication reduces blood levels of vitamin B12, folic acid and sodium; diuretics reduce blood levels of potassium, calcium and vitamin B1 and increase excretion of magnesium and vitamin K; HRT and the oral contraceptive pill cause a reduction in blood levels of vitamins B6 and B12, folic acid and zinc, among others; thyroid hormones cause increased excretion of calcium. These are just some examples of the more common drug–nutrient interactions that we take into account when determining individual supplement programmes.

'Do you think you might be able to help with another problem that I have got?'

At the Clinic we have experience in many diseases, illnesses and disorders. It is often the case that a patient will have various health issues when he or she approaches us for help: for example, high blood pressure, high cholesterol, hormone imbalances – menopause, difficulties with conception, enlarged prostate – psoriasis, depression, panic disorder, thyroid dysfunction, IBS, candida, overweight, underweight, etc. Fundamentally, we guide you as an individual rather than treating the disease.

'I have been doing all that you suggest, including taking supplements, but I don't seem to be getting anywhere'

Some people with arthritic disease have more of a toxin overload than others. If you are struggling to improve, don't be disheartened. Contact us at the Clinic; we will help you think about how this has happened and where you can reduce your exposure to toxins. It is helpful to

- avoid the use of chemicals;
- use the microwave sparingly;
- use a water filter in your kitchen;
- vary the type of fish you eat;
- avoid vaccinations;

- keep six feet (two metres) away from anyone else's mobile phone and use it only on speaker phone;
- turn off WiFi when it is not in use;

and lots more besides . . .

For example, think about

- where you have worked, e.g. an industrial environment, farm or office;
- what sort of environment you have been in for work and your home – e.g. urban or rural;
- the hobbies you have had, e.g. jewellery manufacture, painting;
- dental and beauty treatments you have undergone, e.g. cosmetics, fillings, implants.

Often, toxins build up slowly and over a period of years. The more information you can provide, the better we can guide you.

Contact us

The Margaret Hills Clinic Ltd, 1 Oaks Precinct, Caesar Road, Kenilworth, Warwickshire CV8 1DP

Website: www.margarethillsclinic.com

Tel: 01926 854783

Email: information@margarethillsclinic.com

Fax: 01926 513133

Appendix 2
The research study

A research study was done in 2003 to scientifically investigate the Margaret Hills treatment for arthritis and assess its effectiveness as compared with conventional medical treatment.

The University of Hertfordshire Faculty of Natural Sciences issued ethical approval for the project. A date was randomly set and 300 people on the Margaret Hills Clinic patient database were selected to be studied. To be included in the study, all the patients had to have access to NHS treatment for arthritis and to have begun the Margaret Hills treatment within the previous three years.

The main findings of the research suggested:

- The Margaret Hills Clinic treatment *is effective* in treating arthritis.
- Some patients have impressive improvements after just a few weeks. However, results are not necessarily instant and tend to occur after about 12–18 months of continual treatment.
- Speed of improvement depends on a variety of factors.

The study commenced with a postal questionnaire distributed to the selected 300 patients at the Margaret Hills Clinic. The questionnaire enabled the collection of the patients' personal details, their diagnosis, and the treatment's effectiveness and drawbacks. The study asked patients to rate:

- relief from pain
- perception of cure
- resumption of mobility
- improvement of quality of life.

It is a common misconception that if the arthritis is of a more severe type or has lasted a very long time then supplements and diet will not be a sufficiently aggressive treatment. It may well take longer to rid the body of the acidity that causes arthritis – understandably so – but the Clinic has seen vast improvements and successes among people with rheumatoid arthritis and the less common types of arthritis, as well as osteoarthritis.

The Margaret Hills treatment is not a complementary treatment. It may be used in conjunction with conventional medications and no harm will be done. However, as the anti-arthritis drugs are suppressive, the results of the Margaret Hills treatment would inevitably be delayed and limited, as it is being counteracted.

It is an alternative approach to treating arthritis. This has been well illustrated in the research document on the effectiveness of the treatment.

Stress

The research project found that over three-quarters of all respondents had experienced some form of exceptional stress in the months prior to onset of their arthritis – irrespective of the type of arthritis diagnosed. These stressors may be:

- physical: trauma or an accident;
- emotional: relationship problems, divorce, bereavement;
- mental: exam preparation, long hours at work.

It appears evident that stress may be a trigger factor, and although interesting, no solid conclusions about the link between stress and arthritis can be made as there were no control subjects to compare with.

Figure 1 (overleaf) refers to people who have been taking the Margaret Hills treatment (MH) as well as remaining on medication prescribed by their doctor. It looks at their progress on the treatment compared to patients who have discontinued their prescribed arthritis medication. Scores are shown across all categories.

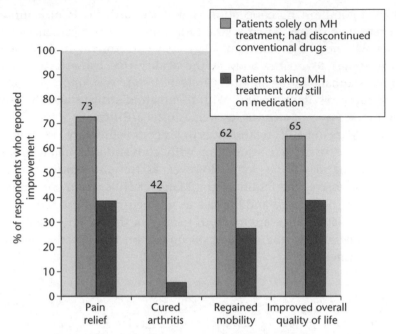

Figure 1 Comparison of effectiveness among those still remaining on prescribed drugs with those who have stopped all arthritis drugs and solely follow the MH programme

Figure 1 clearly displays

- that a far higher percentage of respondents reported improvement across all the categories when they had stopped taking their prescribed medication;
- the limitations of the Margaret Hills treatment when patients remain on their drugs.

Note: It must be impressed that a *gradual* reduction in drugs is required, and if pain persists the Margaret Hills Clinic can propose various ways to overcome this as necessary.

A high number of respondents to the questionnaire (59 per cent) reported experiencing *side-effects with their prescribed medication* that were severe enough to cause them to wish to discontinue the drugs. Side-effects reported by the respondents were nausea and stomach problems, headaches and dizziness, depression and sleeping problems. The second most popular reason was that patients reported their arthritis symptoms still persisting or even getting worse despite taking the medication prescribed. As a consequence of these apparently common circumstances, most of the patients at the first point of contact with the Margaret Hills Clinic are on medication, and sometimes there is quite a long list of their tried and tested drugs! These reported problems highlight the need for a different approach to the treatment of arthritis. The Margaret Hills treatment is a very different approach.

The general outline of the Margaret Hills treatment is to:

- *detoxify* the excess acid state of the body (by drinking well-diluted cider vinegar, taking Epsom salts baths, etc.);
- reduce intake of foods and drinks that have an acidic effect on the body – guidance is given as to what fruits, meats, drinks, etc., to have on the *diet*;
- replenish the *vitamins, minerals, protein* and *trace elements* that are lacking but vitally important for proper functioning of all body systems.

At the Margaret Hills Clinic, the treatment programme includes taking a range of vitamins and minerals. These are formulated in precise quantities as, in order to absorb one nutrient, you need sufficient levels of another. This is important to understand, as if you self-prescribe individual nutrients without the correct guidance, they may be useless and a waste of time and money.

How effective is the Margaret Hills treatment compared to the effectiveness of conventional drugs?

Figure 2 (overleaf) is a graphical display of how the Margaret Hills treatment fares in the category of *pain relief.*

Figure 2 displays the patients' reported pain relief in each group. This shows that more pain relief was experienced when patients had stopped their conventional drugs. The third group reported dramatically *less* pain relief; this group were still taking their conventional medication alongside the Margaret Hills treatment and

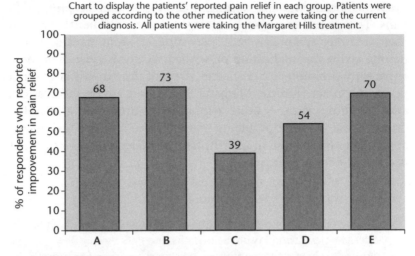

Chart to display the patients' reported pain relief in each group. Patients were grouped according to the other medication they were taking or the current diagnosis. All patients were taking the Margaret Hills treatment.

Figure 2 Perceived pain relief from MH treatment in categories of osteoarthritis, rheumatoid arthritis and other arthritic diseases

A Never taken conventional drugs; **B** discontinued conventional drugs; **C** currently taking conventional drugs; **D** diagnosed with rheumatoid arthritis; **E** diagnosed with ankylosing spondylitis, juvenile arthritis, gout, polymyalgia rheumatica, crystal arthritis

Note: Osteoarthritis, being the most common, has been further subdivided into three categories depending on prescribed medication.

they seemed hindered in their progress. This can be explained by simply looking at the nature of the treatments.

Drugs such as anti-inflammatories are suppressive of the arthritic condition. They can act quite well in relieving pain and other symptoms, but when they are discontinued the arthritis is still there – perhaps even worse. The drugs have been masking the symptoms.

The Margaret Hills treatment acts in a different way: it aims to gradually change the degree of acidity that has built up in the tissues over the years. In this way, the treatment removes the underlying cause of the aches, pains, swellings and stiffness that have been diagnosed as a form of arthritis.

If both treatments are followed then the Margaret Hills treatment has its limitations as this is a 'tug of war' situation.

(Patients must be aware that it may be harmful to discontinue their arthritis medication quickly and without the guidance of a doctor. At the Margaret Hills Clinic, patients are advised to gradually reduce each drug one at a time at a specified reduction in dosage, while always informing their doctor and/or rheumatologist of any changes.)

Rheumatoid arthritis

The group of respondents in the research study diagnosed with rheumatoid arthritis were a particularly interesting group to analyse.

As there are very specific drugs available to target the immune system, an equivalent improvement due to the Margaret Hills treatment was unexpected; theoretically, it wouldn't have the efficacy of these disease-modifying anti-rheumatic drugs (DMARDs).

However, in terms of pain relief and the return of mobility, *both conventional treatment and the Margaret Hills treatment had equal scores for effectiveness.* See Figure 3.

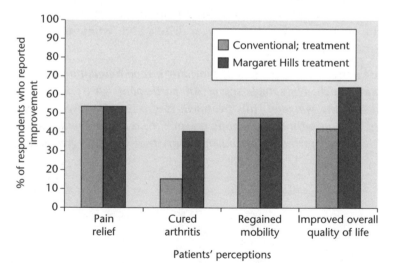

Figure 3 Rheumatoid arthritis – a direct comparison of the perceived effectiveness of conventional medical treatment and MH treatment over all categories

Rheumatoid arthritis (RA) can sometimes be dramatically affected by food, as certain types of RA may be triggered by food allergies. This may explain the improvements as a result of the Margaret Hills acid-free diet. In this same group, 40 per cent of respondents perceived a cure of their RA by the Margaret Hills treatment compared to 15 per cent who attributed their perceived cure to conventional treatment.

> This difference in effectiveness of each treatment was statistically significant in favour of the Margaret Hills treatment. Of all patients, 64 per cent reported an improved quality of life while on the Margaret Hills treatment.

Comment

One of the most important points to understand is that the Margaret Hills Clinic does not expect an individual to improve unless all three aspects of the basic treatment are followed at the same time, i.e.

- the acid-free diet
- the supplementary vitamins, minerals and protein
- the acid-removing cider vinegar drinks and, where possible, the Epsom salts baths.

Please note: This is a pilot study providing a good foundation for possible future research. The sample size of 300 participants gave positive indications that the Margaret Hills treatment is effective. However, it must be noted that, as with any scientific research, in order to produce any concrete evidence, further research is necessary that goes into greater detail.

Index